The Common Sense Guide to Dementia
for Clinicians and Caregivers

Rec'd 9-30-23

Anne M. Lipton • Cindy D. Marshall

The Common Sense Guide to Dementia for Clinicians and Caregivers

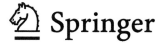 Springer

Anne M. Lipton, M.D., Ph.D.
Diplomate in Neurology
American Board of Psychiatry
  and Neurology

Cindy D. Marshall, M.D.
Director, Memory Center,
  Baylor Neuroscience Center
Baylor University Medical Center
Dallas, TX, USA

ISBN 978-1-4614-4162-5   ISBN 978-1-4614-4163-2 (eBook)
DOI 10.1007/978-1-4614-4163-2
Springer New York Heidelberg Dordrecht London

Library of Congress Control Number: 2012940749

Printed on acid-free paper

Springer is part of Springer Science+Business Media (www.springer.com)

To our patients and families who share their lives and teach us every day.

Foreword

Dr. Robert Katzman of the United States (US) warned in 1976 that, because of the demographic revolution in developed countries of a rapidly aging population, Alzheimer's disease (AD) and other dementing illnesses would soon reign among society's major killers.

His prediction has now been realized. AD now stands as the sixth leading cause of death and the only one among the leading causes of death in the US that lacks truly effective therapies. An estimated 5.3 million Americans have AD (this is almost certainly an underestimate, as many persons with the disorder are not diagnosed) and the Alzheimer's Association estimates that the annual costs of caring for patients with AD has already approached $200 billion. In coming years, the problems will only worsen as the US population continues to age, with the first of the "baby boomers" (people born from 1946 to 1964) now turning 65 and older. AD thus represents a public health problem of enormous proportions.

Although in older adulthood, Alzheimer disease is by far the leading cause of dementia, other non-Alzheimer dementing disorders (e.g., Vascular dementia, Frontotemporal dementia, and Dementia with Lewy bodies) in many respects pose the same challenges and emotional turmoil for caregivers.

It is the human cost of AD and related disorders that is devastating for those with dementia and perhaps even more so for their loved ones. The inevitable deterioration of the defining attributes of individuals that make them uniquely human—memory, language, reasoning, personality—is heart wrenchingly difficult for both patients and caregivers to endure. Over an average duration from symptom onset to death of 7–10 years, AD invariably progressively disables and ultimately results in total dependence. Caring for an individual with AD is associated with "caregiver burden" and deleterious effects on health, income, and fiscal security, as well as the emotional toll of watching the disease rob the very essence of a loved one.

Well-established and helpful sources of information and support exist for caregivers who are facing the problem of dementia in a loved one, including the national Alzheimer's Association (www.alz.org). However, there is also a great need for a comprehensive guide to all the different facets of caregiving that is informative and approachable. We are fortunate that Anne M. Lipton, MD, PhD, and Cindy D. Marshall, MD, have provided this book.

Both Dr. Lipton, a neurologist, and Dr. Marshall, a geriatric psychiatrist, are highly experienced in diagnosing and caring for individuals with Alzheimer disease and other dementing illnesses. In The Common Sense Guide to Dementia, they speak to all caregivers in plain language to educate about important topics. They provide clear definitions of what can be a confusing array of terms associated with the dementing disorders and emphasize their points with case illustrations and common sense rules. Most critically, they remain focused on the practical aspects of caregiving, including how to seek a diagnosis for a loved one, a checklist of what to bring for a visit to the doctor, and very helpful recommendations on how to address such difficult situations as "retiring" a person from driving who is no longer safe to drive. Here also is useful information on nonpharmacological approaches to dementia management, a consideration of end-of-life issues, and how to care for the caregiver.

This Common Sense Guide is directed toward and will indeed benefit all types of caregivers, including health professionals, dealing with AD and other dementias. Drs. Lipton and Marshall clearly wish to help both those affected by dementia and their carers, and we are fortunate that they have provided us with such a useful guide on how to do so with this book.

St. Louis, MO, USA   John C. Morris

Preface

We respect and appreciate patients and all types of caregivers, be they family or friends, professionals or volunteers. That is why we have written a book that can speak to everyone who may play an important part in the care of a patient. Our primary intent is caregiver education, and, as such, our book is specifically designed, written, and addressed to the caregivers of a patient rather than speaking directly to a patient. However, we recognize and respect the fact that some patients with Mild Cognitive Impairment or early-stage dementia may find our observations useful, and we welcome such interest.

Although this book follows a logical order and grouping of caregiving topics, it need not be read from cover to cover. In fact, in our experience, some caregivers might find it overwhelming to do so. Therefore, we have written each chapter so that it may be read on its own, as can individual subheadings. A comprehensive index can be consulted as needed for information on specific topics. We note that the last couple of chapters may be difficult to read for some caregivers, and we recommend reserving reading those until the caregiver is in a good frame of mind and when these chapters have become relevant.

Note on terminology: Please note that we sometimes use the term "doctor" as a convenient shorthand that might apply not only to physicians per se but to any of those who, when and where warranted, may legally and practically fulfill some or all of the "doctor" role, such as explaining diagnosis, providing non-pharmacologic treatment, or even prescribing medications. This may include nurses, nurse practitioners, physician's assistants, medical assistants, psychologists, neuropsychologists, counselors, psychotherapists, occupational therapists, physical therapists, speech therapists/speech-language pathologists, pharmacists, pharmacy technicians, other allied health professionals, and even other medical or office staff, who may often act as an extension ("the ear and the voice") of physicians. Similarly, when we discuss family, we are including any of those nonprofessional but vital caregivers who may have medical Power of Attorney, accompany a patient to a doctor's visit, or perform roles typically performed by a family member, when such a relative is not available.

Texas, USA   Anne M. Lipton, M.D., Ph.D.
                                                                            Cindy D. Marshall, M.D.

Acknowledgments

We are thankful for the opportunity to have worked with so many wonderful patients, families, volunteers, and other caregivers over the years. We are especially grateful for the unwavering support and tolerance of our own families in the writing of this book. We acknowledge the invaluable input of Carol P. Dabner, J.D., Senior Counsel for Underwood Perkins, P.C., in Dallas and a specialist in elder law. We appreciate her expert review of our chapter dealing with legal issues. And, we send a special message of thanks to Rhonda Moore, our long-standing assistant, who is a model of compassion.

Disclosure

Although the case examples stem from our experiences as dementia specialists, any and all private health information has been protected by omitting, altering, or combining as a composite the details of any individual to protect and preserve confidentiality.

Contents

Part II Common Sense Dementia Care

Chapter 1
What Is Dementia?

All Alzheimer's disease is dementia, but not all dementia is Alzheimer's disease. Despite this crucial distinction, even experienced clinicians often confuse these terms. It is important to understand and differentiate the specific type of dementia affecting a patient as the specific diagnosis may determine both treatment and prognosis. And these are usually the overarching concerns of loved ones from the very start of the dementing illness and the clinical evaluation. So—what is dementia? And—what are the signs?

Basic Clinical Definitions

First, let us define some commonly used clinical terms. The clinical term prognosis refers to the expected course of a disease, including the duration or how long it will last. This is usually one of the most important concerns of a patient and his or her family regarding any clinical diagnosis (including dementia). When physicians use the term "progressive or progressing," we are usually referring to the progressive *worsening* of a disease state, unless specifically stated otherwise. We also use the term "onset" to indicate the way a disease starts. An acute onset refers to a disease that presents suddenly over seconds, minutes, hours, or perhaps even a few days. A subacute onset means that a disease presents over days to a few weeks. Illnesses that occur over weeks, months, and years are considered to have a "gradual" onset. The progression of a disease may also be acute, subacute, or gradual. Dementia is therefore usually a disease with gradual onset and progression. Because the symptoms of dementia often begin so subtly and surreptitiously, "sneaking up" on a patient, dementia is often described as having an "insidious" onset.

A.M. Lipton and C.D. Marshall, *The Common Sense Guide to Dementia for Clinicians and Caregivers*, DOI 10.1007/978-1-4614-4163-2_1,
© Springer Science+Business Media, LLC 2013

Table 1.1 Types of onset and progression

	Onset of symptoms	Disease progression
Acute	Days or less	Days or less
Subacute	Days to a few weeks	Days to a few weeks
Gradual	Months or years	Months or years
Stepwise	Acute or gradual	Months or years interspersed with time points of acute worsening which may be followed by stabilization or improvement of acute symptoms

In some cases, fluctuations in the progression may be seen, such that occasional acute worsening or even transient mild improvements may be seen, but a dementia will continue to gradually worsen (progress) over a period of years. Stepwise progression refers to a type of progression that is gradual overall but with time points of acute worsening, sometimes followed by improvement and/or stabilization of the acute symptoms. This may be seen in Vascular dementia in which a patient has acute worsening of cognitive and/or behavioral symptoms each time he or she has a stroke, perhaps followed by some stabilization or even improvement in the new symptoms (but not of the problems preceding the stroke) (Table 1.1).

If symptoms begin or progress (worsen) more suddenly, then an unusual type of dementia or an alternate diagnosis should be considered. Dementia is a terminal illness in that it may eventually result in death in the absence of any other factors. However, many patients with dementia have cardiovascular and other associated disease states. Therefore, patients with dementia may die of cardiovascular (e.g., strokes or heart attacks) or other causes before succumbing to dementia [1].

Dementia: Definitions

Dementia refers to a gradually progressive brain illness that affects cognition (thinking) and/or behavior to such an extent that daily function is impaired. We therefore use the terms dementing illness and dementia interchangeably throughout our text.

Alzheimer's disease (AD) refers to a specific type of dementia in which memory "leads the way" and problems with recall are the "first and worst" issue. Although researchers and medical publications often use the term "Alzheimer disease" for this specific type of dementia, our usage of the possessive term, Alzheimer's disease, reflects the common usage of the general public, clinicians, and residential and support organizations, all of whom comprise the target audience for this book. We also use the abbreviation AD, which is a commonly accepted shorthand for Alzheimer's disease (or Alzheimer disease).

Clinicians use the terms cognition or mental status function, when referring thought processes such as attention and concentration, memory, language, visuospatial skills (which include hand–eye coordination), and complex thought processes known as executive functions. Each of these categories constitutes the so-called cognitive domain. The cognitive domain of *executive functioning* includes those complex thought processes that help us learn in school and perform at work, including sustained attention, planning, organization, judgment, anticipation, ability to alternate between tasks (mental set-shifting), and response inhibition. Synonyms for cognition used in this text include thinking, mentation, mental processes, and mental status function. Formal assessment of these cognitive domains may be done by physicians, neuropsychologists, or others and referred to as mental status testing, neurocognitive evaluation, or neuropsychological testing. Neuropsychological evaluations tend to be the most comprehensive of all of these.

Mood is used clinically to indicate how someone describes his or her own emotional state. Affect is the clinical term referring to how the emotional state of a patient is perceived by the professional evaluator. Psychosis refers to an affective condition in which a patient has lost touch with reality and has hallucinations, delusions, or both. Hallucinations refer to abnormal sensory experiences in which one perceives something that isn't really there. These may be visual (seeing things), auditory (hearing something), or tactile (sensation of feeling something), or affect taste (gustatory) or smell (olfactory). In dementia, visual hallucinations are the most common, but auditory hallucinations may also occur. Tactile hallucinations suggest a different diagnosis than dementia. Delusions designate a mistaken belief, such as believing that another person is present when they are not. Delusions may involve paranoia (in which a patient mistakenly believes that others are trying to inflict harm in some way). The presence of psychosis in the initial months or years of a dementia suggests a non-Alzheimer's dementia.

Onset of Dementia

As noted above, dementia starts gradually and often insidiously, such that the initial symptoms do not cause much concern. Behavioral or cognitive problems that interfere with daily function are not normal. Gradually progressive memory loss is the most common, but by no means the only way in which dementia may begin (see Chap. 2). The initial symptoms should be noted carefully as they often help in making a specific diagnosis. A useful mnemonic (memory device) to recall the major symptom areas involved is to remember the "ABCs" of dementia: *A*ctivities, *B*ehaviors, and *C*ognition.

Progression of Dementia

As specifically applied to dementia, "gradual progression" refers to worsening of the clinical condition over years. A few rare types of dementia can result in more rapid deterioration. However, even in these unusual cases, the initial onset of symptoms usually occurs over months to years (and not over minutes or hours or even days or weeks). By definition, symptoms of dementia must be present for at least 6 months to make a diagnosis. There is no such thing as "rapidly progressive" AD and an alternative or additional diagnosis should be sought if a patient has been diagnosed with AD and the progression of symptoms occurs over fewer than 6 months.

Stages of Care

Different stages of dementing illness have distinctive care requirements. Staging schemes can be useful constructs but serve as guidelines only since dementia progresses uniquely for each individual.

We find the classification of dementia into mild, moderate, severe, and late stages [2] to be the most clinically useful construct and the most practical paradigm for caregivers. A person with a mild dementia may have memory loss (and/or other mild cognitive and/or behavioral deficits) with a few problems in more complex daily functions (or if using the Mild Cognitive Impairment rubric, no such functional deficits). Someone with moderate-stage dementia would have more serious cognitive and/or behavioral deficits along with significant deficits in daily activities and might need some assistance with simple Activities of Daily Living (ADLs), such as eating, dressing, and behavior. A patient with severe dementia has severe cognitive and/or behavioral impairments and needs significant or total assistance with basic tasks. Late-stage dementia denotes the terminal phase of this illness and is discussed in Chap. 16.

We recommend that caregivers retain a general understanding of and plan of care for each of these stages, but focus their attention and efforts in meeting the current and ongoing needs of a loved one with dementia.

References

1. Kukull WA, Brenner DE, Speck CE, Nochlin D, Bowen J, McCormick W, Teri L, Pfanschmidt ML, Larson EB. Causes of death associated with Alzheimer disease: variation by level of cognitive impairment before death. J Am Geriatr Soc. 1994;42(7):723–6.
2. Morris JC. Clinical dementia rating: a reliable and valid diagnostic and staging measure for dementia of the Alzheimer type. Int Psychogeriatr. 1997;9 Suppl 1:173–6. discussion 177–8.

Part I
Start of Care

Chapter 2
Signposts: What to Look for and When to Seek Help

Not knowing is worse than knowing

If you are reading this book, you probably have some knowledge of dementia and its warning signs. However, much more awareness is needed, including in the medical community. Unfortunately, patients are very often not diagnosed with dementia or referred to dementia specialists until 2–3 years after the onset of their symptoms [1]. Not only laypeople, but many medical professionals, continue to hold a mistaken and outmoded viewpoint that nothing can be done for dementia. This nihilism is unwarranted and can even be harmful in delaying or preventing appropriate intervention or resulting in inappropriate or deleterious treatment. Earlier detection of dementia often allays anxieties about unnamed and undiagnosed problems and allows a chance to capitalize on planning, treatment, and research opportunities.

Common sense rule: Most types of dementia are treatable.

Dementias are complex and often require comprehensive evaluation by a specialist (or specialists) for specific diagnosis. This book focuses on finding such an expert and optimal care of a patient already diagnosed with dementia, but, because proper diagnosis is one of the foundations of patient care, it is important to review the basics of what is — and what isn't — indicative of a possible dementia.

A 73 year-old man, who was a retired engineer, was brought to the dementia clinic by his family. He had been having memory problems for 9 months which concerned all of them (patient and family), and his family was also worried that he had become socially withdrawn from interactions with them and others and was much less active than used to be. (Until the last few month, he had golfed several times weekly and attended his grandchildren's ballgames.) He had been diagnosed with "depression" and prescribed alprazolam (trade name: Xanax) twice daily by his primary care physician. He had no prior history of depression and continued with significant memory problems, as well as anxiety, on alprazolam. After a comprehensive assessment, including neuropsychological evaluation and brain MRI, he and his family returned for a follow-up visit. The specialist discussed test results and diagnosis, which was Alzheimer's disease (AD). Although the patient and his

A.M. Lipton and C.D. Marshall, *The Common Sense Guide to Dementia for Clinicians and Caregivers*, DOI 10.1007/978-1-4614-4163-2_2, © Springer Science+Business Media, LLC 2013

family expressed the typical dismay in hearing this diagnosis, all acknowledged that it was a relief to know the reason for his problems. The dementia specialist encouraged resumption of prior activities and directions for tapering off alprazolam over a couple of weeks. At a second follow-up visit, the patient and his family reported that he was not having any anxiety, had resumed his usual social and other activities with his previous level of enthusiasm, and his thinking actually seemed a bit clearer off of the alprazolam. Prescription cognitive enhancers were gradually added over the next few months.

This case points out the sometimes essential role of a dementia specialist in proper diagnosis and treatment of dementia, including selection of medications. In our experience, many well-meaning general practitioners may prescribe medications for dementia symptoms that actually exacerbate memory loss or other problems. We have also found that geographical distance between a patient and family members may be a significantly contributing factor to a family's lack of knowledge regarding a patient's cognitive, behavioral, and functional difficulties. However, case after case has made clear to us that even families who live relatively close by may also lack awareness of such problems or the consequences, including the need for familial, medical, or other intervention. (In fact, because the symptoms occur so slowly and gradually, those closest to the patient may not recognize the problems or how much they have "taken over" for the patient.) Any memory problems that interfere with daily function are not normal and indicate the need for medical attention. Since a patient with such difficulties is unlikely to initiate a medical assessment, it is important for loved ones to recognize and address these issues.

Although memory impairment is the most common presenting symptom of dementing illness, it is by no means the only one. Dementia may begin with changes in a person's cognition, behavior, or function, but it can also begin with motor problems. How a dementia begins is often key to making the diagnosis. This is so important as to reiterate this point: *Knowing the initial signs of a dementia may clinch the diagnosis.* In medical school, we were taught that "the patient makes the diagnosis," meaning that the history of how an illness presents and progresses leads to an answer of what disease process it is. In the case of dementia, it is more often the family that "makes the diagnosis." This is because one of the earliest signs of dementia is loss of insight (loss of awareness) into one's problems, such that sometimes the problem is not even recognized by the patient. Since patients may forget or have unawareness (anosognosia) of details important in discerning the diagnosis, it is crucial for family members to communicate problems to the doctor or other examiner (see Chaps. 4–5 for help with this).

This chapter deals with some specifics of dementia and WHEN medical attention should be sought. The symptoms concerning for dementia are seen in three main areas, which can be thought of as the "ABCs" of dementia: *A*ctivities, *B*ehaviors, and *C*ognition. Memory loss is the most common sign of dementia.

Common sense rule: Memory loss is the most common, but not the only, sign of dementia.

As dementia specialists, we are often asked when medical attention should be sought for memory problems. The first principle is that memory loss that interferes with daily function is not normal. Such memory loss may or may not be related to dementia, but demands medical attention. The same applies to other cognitive or behavioral problems that prevent a person from independently performing his or her usual activities.

Common sense rule: Serious problems should be taken seriously.

Selected Types of Dementia

Not are dementias inherently complex, but every individual has a different onset and course of disease. And, of course, there are exceptions to every rule. We recommend that those interested in more detailed and unusual facets of dementia diagnosis consult the many textbooks (e.g., [2, 3]), articles, and courses devoted to such considerations. We therefore present the following thumbnail sketches of some common dementia types to help in understanding some basic types of common dementias, but, by no means do these brief summaries represent comprehensive diagnostic guidelines.

Alzheimer's Disease

Signs of Alzheimer's Disease

Since Alzheimer's Disease (AD) is the most common and most widely studied dementia, let us begin with it as our archetypal dementia. The six As of Alzheimer's Disease is a useful way to summarize the five areas of cognition that may be impaired as well as to acknowledge that mood and behavior may also be affected [4]. Note the "A" that is not on the list: Attention. This is because simple attention is usually initially well preserved in AD (Table 2.1).

AD is a common disease and the most common form of dementia [5]. Age is usually the greatest risk factor for disease and AD typically affects people aged 65 years and over. Memory is often the "first and worst" problem and is said to "lead the way" in AD. AD usually starts with subtle memory loss and gradually progresses (over years) to affect other cognitive domains, such as language, visuospatial skills, motor skills, executive functioning (e.g., judgment), as well as behavior. Patients with AD

Table 2.1 The six As of Alzheimer's disease

The six As of AD	Common initial symptoms in AD
Amnesia	Forgetful of recent people or events
Agnosia	Difficulty recognizing faces or objects
Aphasia	Problems coming up with names of people or objects
Apraxia	Impaired ability to operate new car, phone, computer, or gadgets
Abstract reasoning	Loss of insight (e.g., reduced awareness of memory problems) (executive functioning)
Affect and behavior	Apathy, social withdrawal

typically have anterograde amnesia or "encoding" memory deficit in which they have significant difficulty learning and remembering information even when given cues (hints or clues). The memory loss usually begins with recent ("short-term") memory, such that the newest information is the hardest to remember. As the disease progresses, remote (or "long-term") memory also starts to fade. To give one example, in the first few years of AD, a patient may start forgetting the names of his or her grandchildren (as these are newer members of the family) and later forget the names of more established family members, such as his or her grown children. Eventually, he or she may confuse present family members for those he or she knew as a child. Another example would be forgetting a recent significant event like a wedding, a party, or a funeral (or the details of such a happening), while still retaining memories from decades ago related to school, family life, work, military service, or social activities. As AD progresses, a patient may tend to dwell in the past and eventually even have difficulty recalling these older ("long-term" or remote) memories.

Mild Cognitive Impairment

Mild Cognitive Impairment (MCI) refers to dementia-type symptoms that are so mild as not to interfere with a person's daily functioning. According to the clinical consensus criteria as set out by a National Institutes of Health expert panel [6], MCI refers to cognitive problems, usually including memory loss, that meet several criteria. The symptoms may be identified by a patient, a family member, or a clinician. The diagnosis should be made clinically, including by formal neurocognitive testing, but may include neuroimaging and additional tests of blood, spinal fluid, etc. A key point in diagnosis of MCI means that a patient retains independence with his or her daily activities and therefore does not meet the criteria for dementia. However, over 5 years, about eight out of ten patients diagnosed with MCI progress or "convert" to a diagnosis of AD (or sometimes other forms of dementia) at a rate of 12–15 %/year [7]. Therefore, MCI usually represents the earliest clinical manifestation of AD [7, 8]. In this book, we generally refer only to dementia, but many of the same issues apply—or may have future application—for patients with MCI and their families.

Besides pure AD, many other kinds of dementia are common. These include Vascular dementia (VaD), Mixed dementia (AD + VaD), Dementia with Lewy bodies (DLB), Parkinson's disease dementia, and Frontotemporal dementia (FTD).

Vascular Dementia

VaD is a dementia caused by one or more infarcts (strokes) in the brain and/or stroke-like changes of small blood vessels (microvascular disease or leukoariaosis) [9]. VaD is also sometimes referred to as Multi-infarct dementia, but since it is not necessary to have *multiple* strokes to incur this diagnosis, we use the more commonly preferred term of VaD. If a patient with VaD has a head MRI or CT, the report of the radiologist may describe microvascular disease as chronic small-vessel ischemic disease or something similar.

The symptoms of VaD may relate to the brain area or areas most affected by vascular disease. Because microvascular disease typically affects the white matter connections of the brain, it interrupts pathways, resulting in slower responses by a patient. You can think of this as "taking the long way home." Thus, this patient eventually arrives at a correct response, but in a more circuitous manner than normal, just as you might have to go a longer way if you were driving and your usual route home was blocked. Similarly, VaD often causes a retrieval memory deficit such that a patient with VaD can recall information if given cues (hints or clues), so their memory is often somewhat better than a patient with AD with an encoding memory deficit (in which the information is not learned and/or stored such that cues do not help). That said, a patient with VaD may have a "retrieval" memory deficit, an encoding memory deficit, or a mixture of these types depending on the areas of the brain affected by vascular disease.

Patients with VaD also often have more striking emotional or "affective" changes than patients with AD. They may also have apathy, depression, agitation, disinhibition (with more impulsive/childlike behavior), personality changes, or a combination of these.

VaD should be considered in patients who have cognitive and/or behavioral problems, particularly those with a history of stroke(s). This may be by history (someone who has had symptoms of a stroke/s) or radiographically (e.g., on head MRI and/or CT). The term "silent" stroke/s refers to an infarct seen on neuroimaging, such as MRI or CT, but with no known clinical symptoms.

In many cases, patients with VaD also have vascular disease elsewhere besides the brain, including the heart (cardiovascular disease) and peripheral vasculature (e.g., peripheral arterial disease). Risk factors for vascular disease associated with VaD include smoking, hypertension (high blood pressure), cholesterol abnormalities (dyslipidemia, hyperlipidemia, hypercholesterolemia), obesity, diabetes, obstructive sleep apnea, and excessive alcohol use. Identifying and treating (or avoiding) these vascular risk factors are crucial in addressing the root problem/s from which VaD stems. They should also be dealt with in other forms of dementias, including AD, to which they also may contribute [10].

VaD may have a more indolent (slower) course than does AD, but the patient's overall course is highly dependent upon the number and extent of vascular risk factors. If these can be minimized, then the prognosis may improve. If the vascular risk factors continue—or worsen—the patients' overall vascular status, including their cerebrovascular function, will most likely decline. The progression of VaD also differs from AD in that it may be stepwise (with sudden decrements followed by periods of plateau/stabilization) representing time points at which strokes occur. Some recovery of acute symptoms may even occur, but the overall course is one of gradual worsening.

Mixed Dementia

Mixed dementia is not a mixture of any old type of dementia but refers to the specific combination of Alzheimer disease and VaD. As one might expect, the symptoms, course, prognosis, and duration are thus a blend of these two dementias and vary based on the degree of each involved. Here again, optimizing the treatment of any vascular risk factors can affect the patient's overall health as well as the course of his or her dementing illness.

Parkinson's Disease Dementia

The cardinal signs of Parkinson's disease (PD) are rest tremor, bradykinesia (slowed movements), rigidity, and postural instability (tendency to fall backwards). These motor symptoms typically respond to treatment with antiparkinsonian medications and progress very slowly (over decades). Some 20 % of patients have cognitive deficits in the early stages of PD and round 30–50 % of patients with Parkinson's disease develop dementia but this usually occurs at a relatively late stage of the disease [11]. The cognitive symptoms of PD tend to differ from AD in that they often include bradyphrenia (slowed thinking), as well as impairments of attention and a retrieval memory deficit (rather than the typical encoding memory deficit of AD) [12].

Parkinson's-Plus Syndromes

These include DLB (also called Lewy body dementia or Lewy body disease), Progressive Supranuclear Palsy (PSP), Motor system atrophy (also known as Shy–Drager disease), and Striatonigral degeneration. Patients with any of these syndromes have parkinsonism with some, but not all, of the cardinal motor features of PD. They also often have other symptoms distinguishing them from pure PD. Moreover, Parkinson's-plus syndromes do not tend to respond (or at least not as robustly) to antiparkinsonian medication. Therefore, they often progress over a few years (rather than over decades as is typically the case for PD).

DLB deserves mention as it is a common cause of dementia. DLB refers to a combination of dementia, parkinsonism (Parkinson-type symptoms), psychosis (usually vivid visual hallucinations, but delusions and other types of hallucinations may occur), and cognitive fluctuations, all transpiring within just a few years (usually less than three) [13]. Patients with DLB tend to have cognitive and behavioral symptoms similar to those seen in Parkinson's disease dementia but these progress more rapidly. The motor symptoms of DLB are often initially less extensive than those of Parkinson's disease (and tremor may be lacking), but do not usually respond as well to antiparkinsonian medications and tend to progress over just a few years (rather than over decades for Parkinson's disease).

More information is available through the American Parkinson's Disease Association at www.apdaparkinson.org and www.lbda.org, the Website for the Lewy Body Dementia Association.

Frontotemporal Dementia

FTD is a disease that typically affects people under the age of 65, especially in their fifties or sixties, and may even be the most common dementia in this age group [14–16]. Like AD, gradual onset and progression are typical. Unlike AD, in which memory loss is the most prominent symptom, the first dementia symptoms in FTD are typically language or behavioral problems [17–19]. Thus, this disease may first be misdiagnosed as a stroke with aphasia or a psychiatric illness (such as depression or bipolar disorder) in a patient with no prior psychiatric history. Patients may also present with motor symptoms, such as weakness or Parkinson's-type symptoms (parkinsonism). The patient's age as well as the onset, course, and associated signs and symptoms are keys to the disease and careful neurological work-up is important in making the correct diagnosis, addressing any motor aspects of this disease, pointing the way to appropriate treatment, and helping to avoid unnecessary, futile, or even harmful evaluations or treatments. The clinical presentation (as well as the pathology) of PSP and FTD overlap, so PSP may present with FTD and parkinsonism may later develop, or vice versa.

Helpful Websites for FTD include:

The Association for Frontotemporal Dementia: www.theaftd.org
Northwestern University Feinberg School of Medicine Cognitive Neurology & Alzheimer's Disease Center www.brain.northwestern.edu
University of California, San Francisco Memory Clinic: www.memory.ucsf.edu

There are many, many other types of dementia and if you are concerned for a patient or a loved one who doesn't have the typical onset and course of AD as outlined below, evaluation by dementia specialist, in conjunction with good primary medical care, may be imperative to identify alternate causes. If you are concerned about a type of dementia not specifically listed here, you can consult with your medical professional/s, as well as books, associations, and Websites dedicated to specific forms of dementia. The National Institutes of Health A–Z list of diseases is especially helpful and can be found at www.nih.gov. And, keep reading, the following chapters are meant to help professional and family caregivers of patients with dementia—no matter what the type.

Traumatic Brain Injury

Traumatic Brain Injury (TBI) is a complex subject since each trauma leaves its own distinct signature and may be affected by age, preexisting trauma, or other medical issues. Besides the type, location, and extent of any given injury (including any loss of consciousness), repetition of brain trauma may contribute to cognitive and behavioral deficits. TBI may result from many causes, including deprivation of oxygen to the brain. Brain injury, particularly repeated trauma with extended loss of consciousness, can also predispose to the development of dementia [20]. Repeated sporting-related head trauma has been linked with Chronic Traumatic Encephalopathy [21]. (Encephalopathy refers to cognitive and behavioral impairments which are permanent and may be progressive.)

Other Diagnostic Considerations

In discussing what dementia is, it is also important to consider what is *not* dementia. Before making a diagnosis of MCI or dementia for a patient with gradual cognitive and/or behavioral decline, a medical work-up should be done to evaluate for other possible primary or contributing causes. Potential etiologies may include depression, thyroid problems, alcohol dependence, certain medications, B12 deficiency, obstructive sleep apnea, and neurosyphilis. All may be treatable to some extent.

Dementia is typically not a "fast" process, but one that occurs gradually over a period of years (even the so-called rapidly progressive dementia, which is rare, occurs over months to years). If mental processes deteriorate (or seem to) at a faster rate (than years), this generally indicates one of several possibilities:

One, the cause is not dementia, but something else, such as a delirium, which can cause mental status changes over a period of hours. As a general rule, the rate of the deterioration is directly proportional to the speed to which one should seek medical attention. That is, the more abrupt the change, the sooner that professional evaluation should be sought. Causes of delirium include head/brain injury, stroke, seizure, infection, alcohol, and drug effect (this can include legal medication taken in recommended dosages). If a person's mentation changes over a period of hours (or shorter), this suggests a serious medical cause, but because of the potential for reversibility, if the cause can be properly identified and treated in a timely fashion, the need for immediate medical attention is underscored.

Of course, a delirium may be superimposed upon a dementia. This often makes diagnosis of dementia in the acute situation difficult, if not impossible, as any delirium must be addressed first and may obscure (and/or exacerbate) an underlying dementia. Diagnosis of an underlying dementing process may be made tentatively or even deferred until resolution of a delirium. It is also important to stress that patients with dementia may have delirium (and are in fact at higher risk for it) and the presence of a dementing illness may obscure diagnosis of an accompanying delirium. For a patient with a previously diagnosed dementia, it is important for those who know the person well, including family and professional care providers, to note sudden changes in thinking, behavior, or daily function. Furthermore, family members and others should emphasize these changes and act as the patient's advocate in asserting the need for medical intervention, even in a medical setting. In our experience as dementia specialists, those who do not know the patient well, including health care professionals, may minimize such mental status alterations in a patient with a prior diagnosis of dementia:

An 82 year-old woman with Alzheimer's disease was living at home with her family. They noted her to have increased confusion with sudden interruption in conversation for several minutes two nights in a row. The first evening, the family had brought the patient to an urgent care clinic and were told that "Oh, she just has dementia" and they should expect her to behave this way as she was "sundowning." However, this was such a marked change from her usual behavior that, when it happened again, they brought her to the emergency department of a local hospital. A doctor there noted that the patient appeared to be having possible visual hallucinations and kept looking to the right. The doctor discussed this with her family who said that they had never noticed her to have such symptoms before. The doctor suspected that something like a stroke or infection which might be causing this, but a CT scan of her head and tests of blood and urine were normal. The doctor then called the patient's neurologist who also indicated that the patient had no history of hallucinations, but that she did have a similar episode of confusion and decreased responsiveness a month prior. An outpatient electroencephalogram (EEG) had been done around that time, but did not show any abnormal epileptiform activity that would suggest a seizure. However, both the neurologist and emergency physician agreed that the patient's history was now even more concerning for possible seizures and that these might be captured on an EEG while the patient was having such symptoms. Therefore, an EEG was performed in the emergency department. The patient was found to have abnormal epileptiform activity consistent with seizure. She was started on seizure medication, her symptoms resolved, and she did not have any further spells. Her family and neurologist agreed that her behavior had also returned to her usual baseline (i.e., what was normal for her) after starting such medicine.

In such a scenario, it is extremely helpful to consult with the patient's usual medical team for input into the alteration from their usual medical condition. And family members shouldn't assume that hospital personnel, either in the emergency department or elsewhere, will automatically contact a patient's primary care provider or specialist.

We recommend that family members not only request emergency or other hospital personnel to inform a patient's existing medical providers of admission (to the Emergency Department and/or hospital), but that the family also call the patient's usual medical team to ensure that they are informed of the patient's situation. We believe that any good primary care physician wants to know when and why one of their patients has to go to the hospital and that any dementia specialist following the patient does as well, whether to provide professional medical history/records for the patient and their hospital team, make medication recommendations, visit the patient, or to provide information for the patient's medical record and follow-up care regarding changes in clinical course, hospital evaluation, and/or any medication reactions. Someone, be it a family member and/or medical professional, who is familiar with a patient's history can make all the difference in advocating for the patient's best interests and helping secure the most appropriate medical care.

Another explanation for cognitive decline in dementia that is faster than expected is that a person with a dementing illness may have "unmasking" of the disease due to a stressor (and more often, multiple stressors) which makes the onset appear more abrupt than it actually is. In our clinical practice, the most common stressors are hospitalization, surgery (whether or not hospitalization is involved), death of a spouse or other caregiver, and/or a move. Hospitalization often involves a number of stressors, including being away from one's home, family/caregiver, and daily routine; pain; illness; addition or alteration of medications; as well as surgical and/or other medical procedures, invasive or otherwise. A person with dementia may function well in his or her own environment, but be extremely vulnerable to decompensation, which serves to make the change in his or her mental status appear much more abrupt than it actually is.

> A 74 year-old man who lived alone was admitted to a Veterans' Affairs hospital with gastric distress and underwent various gastric procedures. He was issued the standard hospital hygiene kit, but seemed befuddled as to how to perform basic Activities of Daily Living (ADLs), such as shaving. His family was consulted and they reported that he had no problems living independently, including using the shaver that he had kept in the same location on his bathroom shelf "for 40 years."

Another possibility is that a patient's history is unknown, not well known, or not recognized as a problem until the occurrence of a significant crisis.

> A 78 year-old woman who lived alone was admitted to a geriatric medical floor for correction of dehydration after she was found on the floor by her family after she had a fall. Her geriatric team requested consultation from a dementia specialist after the patient persisted with cognitive problems even after her dehydration was corrected and no other significant medical problems were found. The geriatric team had spoken with the family who confirmed that the patient lived alone and "independently." The dementia specialist evaluated the patient and found her to have excellent attention (which is usually impaired in cases of delirium) but moderate-to-severe impairments of memory and executive functioning. The specialist obtained new history from the family which indicated that the patient didn't drive and that, over the last year, they had assumed management of her finances and done all of her grocery shopping and some of her housekeeping.

Summary

The main aspects, or "ABCs," of dementia are Activities, Behaviors, and Cognition. Memory loss is the most common sign of dementia, but there are many types of dementia and even the same type of dementia may differ in presentation among individual patients. While dementias are generally not curable, and few are reversible, such illnesses often can be treated to some extent. It is important to identify and treat any other medical conditions, such as delirium, which may worsen or mimic a dementia. If this chapter has helped you decide that you do, in fact, need to get help for someone with dementia, the next chapter will guide you on the how-to of finding it.

Websites

Alzheimer's Association: www.alz.org
American Parkinson's Disease Association: www.apdaparkinson.org
Lewy Body Dementia Association: www.lbda.org
Association for Frontotemporal Dementia: www.theaftd.org
Northwestern University Feinberg School of Medicine Cognitive Neurology &
Alzheimer's Disease Center www.brain.northwestern.edu
University of California, San Francisco Memory Clinic: www.memory.ucsf.edu
The National Institutes of Health: www.nih.gov

Common Sense Rules

- Most types of dementia are treatable.
- Memory loss is the most common, but not the only, sign of dementia.
- Serious problems should be taken seriously.

References

1. Jost BC, Grossberg GT. The natural history of Alzheimer's disease: a brain bank study. J Am Geriatr Soc. 1995;43(11):1248–55.
2. Weiner MF, Lipton AM, editors. The American Psychiatric Publishing Textbook of Alzheimer Disease and Other Dementias. Washington, DC: American Psychiatric Publishing, Inc.; 2009.
3. Weiner MF, Lipton AM, editors. Clinical Manual of Alzheimer disease and other Dementias. Washington, DC: American Psychiatric Publishing, Inc.; 2012.
4. McKhann GM, Knopman DS, Chertkow H, Hyman BT, Jack Jr CR, Kawas CH, et al. The diagnosis of dementia due to Alzheimer's disease: recommendations from the National Institute on Aging and the Alzheimer's Association workgroup. Alzheimers Dement. 2011;7(3):263–9.
5. Morris JC. Differential diagnosis of Alzheimer's disease. Clin Geriatr Med. 1994;10(2):257–76.
6. Albert M, DeKosky ST, Dickson D, Dubois B, Feldman H, Fox NC, et al. The diagnosis of mild cognitive impairment due to Alzheimer's disease: report of the National Institute on Aging and the Alzheimer'sAssociation workgroup. Alzheimers Dement. 2011;7(3):270–9.
7. Petersen RC. Conversion. Neurology. 2006;67:S12–3.
8. Morris JC. Mild cognitive impairment is early-stage Alzheimer disease: time to revise diagnostic criteria. Arch Neurol. 2006;63:15–6.
9. Roman GC, Tatemichi TK, Erkinjuntti T, Cummings JL, Masdeu JC, Garcia JH, et al. Vascular dementia: diagnostic criteria for research studies: report of the NINDS-AIREN International Workshop. Neurology. 1993;43:250–60.
10. Debette S, Seshadri S, Beiser A, Au R, Himali JJ, Palumbo C, Wolf PA, Decarli C. Midlife vascular risk factor exposure accelerates structural brain aging and cognitive decline. Neurology. 2011;77(5):461–8.
11. Aarsland D, Zaccai J, Brayne C. A systematic review of prevalence studies of dementia in Parkinson's disease. Mov Disord. 2005;20:1255–63.

12. Aarsland D, Andersen K, Larsen JP, Lolk A. Prevalence and characteristics of dementia in Parkinson disease: an 8-year prospective study. Arch Neurol. 2003;60:387–92.
13. McKeith IG, Dickson DW, Lowe J, Emre M, O'Brien JT, Feldman H, et al. Diagnosis and management of dementia with Lewy bodies: third report of the DLB Consortium. Neurology. 2005;65:1863–72.
14. Knopman DS, Petersen RC, Edland SD, et al. The incidence of frontotemporal lobar degeneration in Rochester, Minnesota, 1990 through 1994. Neurology. 2004;62:506–8.
15. Ratnavalli E, Brayne C, Dawson K, Hodges JR. The prevalence of frontotemporal dementia. Neurology. 2002;58:1615–21.
16. Rosso SM, Donker Kaat L, Baks T, et al. Frontotemporal dementia in The Netherlands: patient characteristics and prevalence estimates from a population-based study. Brain. 2003;126: 2016–22.
17. Neary D, Snowden JS, Gustafson L, Passant U, Stuss D, Black S, et al. Frontotemporal lobar degeneration: a consensus on clinical diagnostic criteria. Neurology. 1998;51:1546–54.
18. McKhann GM, Albert MS, Grossman M, Miller B, Dickson D, Trojanowski JQ. Clinical and pathological diagnosis of frontotemporal dementia: report of the Work Group on Frontotemporal Dementia and Pick's Disease. Arch Neurol. 2001;58:1803–9.
19. Rascovsky K, Hodges JR, Kipps CM, Johnson JK, Seeley WW, Mendez MF, et al. Diagnostic criteria for the behavioral variant of frontotemporal dementia (bvFTD): current limitations and future directions. Alzheimer Dis Assoc Disord. 2007;21:S14–8.
20. Mehta KM, Ott A, Kalmijn S, Slooter AJ, van Duijn CM, Hofman A, Breteler MM. Head trauma and risk of dementia and Alzheimer's disease: the Rotterdam Study. Neurology. 1999;53(9):1959–62.
21. Omalu B, Bailes J, Hamilton RL, Kamboh MI, Hammers J, Case M, Fitzsimmons R. Emerging histomorphologic phenotypes of chronic traumatic encephalopathy in American athletes. Neurosurgery. 2011;69(1):173–83.

Chapter 3
Finding Help

"A journey of a thousand miles begins with a single step."
—Lao Tzu

Chapter 2 dealt with when help should be sought on the basis of symptoms of dementia. This chapter addresses how and where to find the right type of assistance and the important role of family members (or their surrogates), in conjunction with medical professionals, on this quest for the right diagnosis, treatment, and additional support.

The major actions involved in procuring such help are (1) advocating for the person with dementia; (2) identifying a physician/s who can provide appropriate assessment, diagnosis, and plan (and accompanying the patient to visits with said doctor/s); and (3) seeking additional resources for the patient and for the caregiver. If you are reading this book, you have already taken an important first step.

Advocating for the Person with Dementia

This section is primarily intended for family members and/or those with medical power of attorney (POA) for patients with warning signs of dementia. However, it may also provide valuable guidance for professionals to keep in mind as they assist patients and families.

If you are concerned that your loved one has dementia, then the ball has landed squarely in your court. Someone with cognitive and/or behavioral impairments may have difficulty arriving at appropriate medical care on his or her own and deserves an advocate towards this goal. Someone with dementia often lacks full awareness of his or her condition and won't seek help on his or her own. A person with dementia also doesn't generally bring cognitive or behavioral symptoms to the attention of his or her primary care physician. In addition, most general practitioners don't routinely screen for dementia. Therefore, it is up to a family member (or surrogate)

A.M. Lipton and C.D. Marshall, *The Common Sense Guide to Dementia for Clinicians and Caregivers*, DOI 10.1007/978-1-4614-4163-2_3, © Springer Science+Business Media, LLC 2013

to support the patient in obtaining the proper evaluation, diagnosis, and treatment. In practical terms, this usually means that a family member must find a doctor (or doctors) to carry out such assessment and management.

One of the most important things that you can do for a family member with dementia or suspected dementia is to attend his or her doctors' visits. This means that you (or your surrogate) should not just wait in the waiting room. We should all be so lucky. A doctor's office can be stressful on a good day, and often we are there when we are at our sickest and most vulnerable. Having a medical partner attend physician visits is a good idea for everyone, but particularly so in the case of someone with possible dementia. Someone who has memory problems may forget to relate certain information and this could be serious if he or she forgets important elements of his or her medical history, such as allergies. Also recall that patients with dementia may lack insight or awareness of their problems and physicians may not learn about cognitive deficits unless they specifically screen for them (and most doctors don't routinely do so). Patients with memory loss due to AD have the most difficulty learning and recalling novel information and this would include any new diagnosis or newly prescribed medications.

Common sense rule: Someone with memory problems (or similar) should not go to the doctor alone.

In the case of physical examinations, the patient, doctor, and family member should work together to decide on the best plan. For patients with moderate-to-severe dementia, it may actually be more reassuring for the patient to have a familiar family member in the room than to be alone. It may also be helpful for a family member/medical POA to witness medical exams or procedures to assess a patient's stress level and help decide when it is no longer worthwhile to continue or repeat evaluations, particularly invasive ones like gynecological exams.

One of the other important functions of a family medical advocate is to call a stop to screening invasive and/or potentially painful examinations and procedures when dementia progresses to a severe stage. Three important questions to ask before an examination or procedure: Do the risks (e.g., the pain or distress from an examination or procedure) outweigh potential benefit/s? Will the evaluation change the patient's management/treatment? Can it help improve the patient's quality of life? For example, it may not be necessary to continue screening mammography, colonoscopy, or lab tests if these are difficult and/or will not change what is being done for a patient with severe dementia. If it is clear that a patient with severe dementia would not be subjected to any surgical biopsy, lumpectomy, or other procedure for a breast lump, no matter how suspicious, then there is no point in continuing to perform (and pay for) mammograms. The patient, family, and community would be far better served by placing time, effort, and finances towards optimizing a patient's quality of life. Another important example is avoiding the placement of a feeding tube for a patient with severe dementia as this has not been shown to be beneficial [1–3], but, unfortunately, continues to be done, sometimes with little or no input from a patient's family [4]. If a doctor or a health care team fails to bring up these issues, a family member or medical POA should raise them. It's often hard for doctors and families NOT to do an exam or procedure. It's hard to say no. But it can be much easier—and kinder—to refuse a test or procedure than to deal with an abnormal result—or an adverse outcome.

Common sense rule: A good advocate may have to speak out and—know when to say no.

As noted above, to be a credible advocate, you have to be there. It takes at least two to diagnose dementia. Most often information from a family member is necessary in making the diagnosis. But what if you live far away or can't attend doctors' visits for another reason? Then, before you find a specialist for the patient, you first need to find someone to act as the patient's advocate in your stead.

If family members/medical POA are not available due to constraints of time, geography, their own health issues, or other reasons, they should enlist the help of others, including other family members and/or a professional caregiver. A geriatric care manager is usually the best bet for faraway families and can be found via the Internet (e.g., the National Association of Professional Geriatric Care Managers Website: www.caremanager.org) and area agencies on aging. A geriatric professional care manager can perform a home evaluation to assess a patient's needs, arrange doctors' appointments and accompany the patient to these, and assist in many other ways (although they require payment for their services).

A professional health aide or similar caregiver hired privately or from a home health agency may be able to help a patient in a variety of ways, including accompanying patients to doctors' visits. A home health agency may perform a needs assessment; however, this is typically not as comprehensive as that of a geriatric care manager. A private nurse is usually the most expensive option, but could certainly apply his or her professional expertise to advantage in a clinical setting.

All professionals should be vetted for prior experience with geriatric and dementia patients. Certifications, references, and recommendations should be sought, including from doctors, other medical personnel, and organizations like your local Alzheimer's Association chapter, as well as friends and family. Do a background check or confirm that one has been done (as is typically the case for employees of a home health agency).

If it is not possible for a family or professional caregiver to attend doctors' visits, close friends, neighbors, housekeepers, and/or coworkers may have to step in. It is helpful if such intermediaries have the support of any next-of-kin. This may include forms designating medical POA, contact information for family members, and/or a brief letter from a family member outlining the situation. Be advised that only the patient can designate a POA. Laws vary from state to state, but generally speaking, a person with the ability to understand such designation may name a durable medical POA to speak for him or her. Therefore, a patient with dementia may be able to designate POA in the earlier stages of dementia, but not in the later stages. Once a patient's dementia is severe enough to impair his or her understanding and judgment, a POA can no longer be designated. In this case, the next-of-kin must substitute judgment. This must be a living relative. The spouse would be considered the first next-of-kin, then parents, any adult children next, then any brothers or sisters, and so on. Unfortunately, in the case of multiple parties sharing equal decision-making power (e.g., more than one child), conflicts may arise, sometimes necessitating costly legal proceedings, even guardianship proceedings, which may cost tens of thousands of dollars. Avoiding the heartaches, headaches, and other costs of family disagreements represent some of the many important reasons why everyone of legal age should designate a durable medical POA (and legal/financial POA as well) (also see Chap. 14).

Some doctors will allow for phone-conferencing during a patient appointment (this is usually most practicable during discussion of diagnosis, etc., rather than during the history or physical examination portions of the visit) or at another scheduled time (usually at an additional cost since most insurance plans, including Medicare, do not reimburse for this).

So now you know that you (or another responsible party) need to go to the doctor with your loved one. But, first you have to find the right doctor.

Primary Medical Care

Once a problem of possible dementia has been identified by someone like a family member or a primary care practitioner, one of the important first steps is to find a medical professional knowledgeable in evaluating and treating this disease, just as one would for any major health problem, such as heart disease or pain.

Fortunately, nowadays, most people have access to a variety of resources to find such specialist. On the other hand, such specialists are often few and far between, especially in rural areas.

If symptoms occur rapidly (over hours or more quickly), emergency medical attention should be sought as this is unlikely to be dementia (it could be delirium or another problem superimposed on dementia).

If symptoms occur gradually, the first point-of-care should be the patient's primary care physician. If the patient does not have one, this is a significant deficit in the patient's health care and a primary care provider should be sought to address any and all medical issues, possibly including dementia, prior to a consultation with a dementia specialist. It is important that medical conditions, including cardiovascular (such as high blood pressure, high cholesterol), endocrine (diabetes and thyroid problems), and pulmonary/respiratory conditions (such as sleep apnea or chronic obstructive pulmonary disease) be addressed, as these may cause or contribute to cognitive problems.

Common sense rule: Everyone should have a primary care physician.

A primary care physician may be qualified, willing, and able to diagnose and manage dementia, but, unfortunately, all too many cases of dementia go undiagnosed and untreated, as has been documented for AD [5]. General practitioners can certainly address dementia, but they often do not have the time and it may not be given a high priority due to the plethora of other medical issues that must be addressed for a single patient. Therefore, we strongly recommend consideration of a referral to a dementia specialist and/or center or clinic.

That said, it is usually worthwhile to first visit with a patient's family doctor to discuss symptoms concerning for dementia and the best plan of action for the patient, including any primary medical work-up, such as blood tests, that should be done. Make sure to ask the primary care doctor for his or her expert recommendation regarding the best specialist dementia doctor/s in the patient's geographic area and a referral to one of these. The primary care doctor may be relieved to have such expert support as dementia typically involves complex and time-consuming evaluation and counseling. If this doctor doesn't have a recommendation, the next section will help you find a dementia expert or a clinic.

Common sense rule: See the primary medical doctor first.

Identifying a Specialist

Who Are Specialists?

Dementia specialists go by a number of titles and specialties. The authors of this book are a geriatric psychiatrist (CM) and behavioral neurologist (AL). These represent subspecialties of psychiatry and neurology, respectively. Medical doctors specializing in dementia include psychiatrists (especially geriatric psychiatrists), neurologists (especially behavioral neurologists and geriatric neurologists), and geriatricians. These doctors may have a doctorate in medicine (M.D.) or Osteopathy (D.O.) and are qualified to diagnose medical illness and prescribe medications. Other professionals, such as psychologists, neuropsychologists, geriatric and psychiatric nurses, nurse practitioners, and physician assistants, may also play an integral role in the evaluation and treatment of dementia, often in concert with physicians.

Neurologists and psychiatrists are medical doctors (M.D. or D.O.). After medical school, they complete a 1-year medical internship and 3 years of residency in their specialty. Neurologists diagnose and treat diseases of the entire nervous system, including the brain. There is often confusion between what psychiatrists and psychologists are and do, so let us make that clear: Psychiatrists diagnose and treat mental illness. Such treatment may include medication and psychotherapy ("talk therapy"). Psychologists also assess mental health and provide invaluable services in the form of psychotherapy and neuropsychological testing. However, a psychologist earns Doctor of Philosophy degree (Ph.D.) which does not allow for the prescribing of medication in most states.

Psychotherapy can be especially valuable for caregivers, but it may be limited or pose special challenges for patients with dementia, who may lack the insight (awareness of their problems) necessary for such therapy. Nevertheless, patients, as well as caregivers, may certainly benefit and its merit should be judged on an individual— and ongoing—basis.

Neuropsychologists are specially trained psychologists who perform and interpret psychometric assessments, such as Intelligence Quotient (IQ) tests, in which cognitive abilities are scored. A comprehensive neuropsychological evaluation includes the administration and scoring of a panel of such tests along with an interpretation of the results. The technical expertise and opinion of a neuropsychologist may be helpful, or even essential, in the evaluation of dementia, especially in complex or unusual cases of dementia, mild cognitive changes, and/or evaluation of capacity (discussed further in Chap. 14).

Neurologists and psychiatrists have training in the evaluation and treatment of dementia, but this varies and should be verified, as should board-certification. In the United States, psychiatrists and neurologists may earn board-certification from the American Board of Psychiatry and Neurology by completing a residency in their field and passing a specialty board examination. Such doctors are considered "general" neurologists or psychiatrists. Some neurologists and psychiatrists also pursue additional training and/or certification in a specific aspect ("subspecialty") of their field. Such subspecialty certification usually entails an additional 1–2 years of fellowship training as well as passing a written subspecialty examination. Doctors in subspecialties of Geriatric Psychiatry, Geriatric Neurology, or Behavioral Neurology have additional training in dementia, but are few and far between, so you are in luck if you find one. Most practice at academic medical centers, such as medical schools.

General neurologists and psychiatrists are typically familiar with diagnosing and treating dementia. Psychiatrists have additional training in the management of behavioral and psychosocial issues, whereas neurologists have special expertise in addressing motor and mobility issues (e.g., weakness, falls) and stroke risk factors and complications. If you are lucky enough to have a choice of specialists, focus on problems which are the worst. A patient with dementia might be evaluated and treated by a psychiatrist or a neurologist. But, one who has irritability might be better served by a psychiatrist, whereas one who has difficulty walking might benefit more from a neurological evaluation. In some cases, it may be helpful to have the two specialists work together. For example, in the case of Parkinson's disease dementia or DLB, a neurologist may attend to the patient's motor symptoms, while a psychiatrist might treat the patient's hallucinations.

A geriatrician is a primary care physician who has additional training and certification in the treatment of patients 65 years and older. Because age is a major risk factor for dementia, it is a disease commonly seen in the elderly, so geriatricians, by definition, usually have a great deal of experience with dementia. They are expert at carefully shepherding the care of patients with advanced dementia to optimize quality of life and avoid unnecessary, expensive, and potentially harmful exams and procedures. On the other hand, if their time and attention must necessarily focus on the management of significant medical issues other than dementia, a referral to another specialist, such as a neurologist or a psychiatrist, may help everyone—the patient, the family, and the doctor.

Common sense rule: Experience and training are more important than title.

Why Consult a Specialist?

An evaluation by a dementia expert helps ensure proper diagnosis and treatment and referral for appropriate research opportunities, as warranted. The earlier in the disease course a patient has such an assessment, the better in terms of optimizing diagnosis (it is easier to make a specific diagnosis before the disease progresses as initial symptoms are key in making this determination), management (including future planning), and prospects for participation in research studies. On the other hand, there is a shortage of such specialists and the time, money, and other effort required if one can be located may be prohibitive. One option is for a patient to have a one-time consultation with a dementia specialist who can send a diagnostic report and recommendations to the patient's general practitioner, who can then follow up on these. While it is not necessary for every patient with suspected dementia to see a specialist, we highly recommend at least one consultation with such an expert when a patient has unusual symptoms (e.g., early hallucinations or motor symptoms), onset (e.g., before age 65), or course (e.g., progression is more rapid than months-to-years).

Common sense rule: Unusual medical cases deserve the attention of a specialist.

How and Where Can I Find a Specialist and Other Resources?

As discussed above, the first and best step in finding a specialist is to obtain a referral for one from the patient's family physician. However, it may be worthwhile to obtain recommendations from other sources as well. You might ask a patient's other doctors, other doctors in the patient's locale, your own doctors, and other medical professionals (do not underestimate the knowledge base of medical office staff who are usually well acquainted with local doctors). Word of mouth from others in your shoes (family, friends, and neighbors) can also be very helpful, although their knowledge of medical professionals may be limited to personal experience.

Because there is a desperate shortage of geriatric psychiatrists, it may be difficult to find one. The American Association for Geriatric Psychiatry (AAGP) provides valuable information for patients and families on their Website (www.aagponline. org), including a search engine to find a geriatric psychiatrist in your area.

A list of National Institutes of Health (NIH) Alzheimer's Disease Centers may be found online at http://www.nia.nih.gov/Alzheimers/ or by calling 1-800-438-4380. These centers generally offer a number of qualified specialists and other support, as well as research opportunities. Once even a tentative dementia diagnosis is made, we recommend consulting the A–Z listing of diseases at the NIH Website (www.nih. gov) and finding the patient information and national support group for that particular disease. The Alzheimer's Association (www.alz.org, telephone help line: 1-800-272-3900) and its local chapters can help locate specialists and also provide a variety of other resources regarding all types of dementia. You can also sign up for their electronic newsletter. Depending on the type of dementia, other local and national support groups, such as the Association for FTD (www.theaftd.org), and the Lewy Body Dementia Association (www.lbda.org), may be beneficial. Attending a caregiver support group, class, course, or symposium may be a great source of information and networking, even (and perhaps especially) during the breaks. In between sessions, take the opportunity to meet and talk to professionals and nonprofessional caregivers alike and benefit from their experiences and suggestions. A number of other caregiver Websites including www.caring.com may assist you. You can set up Google alerts for news on dementia and/or a specific type of dementia to receive updates on these topics. A significant method of helping someone with dementia is to educate yourself. If you don't use a computer, try reading books such as this one, calling one or more of the organizations listed above, and visiting their local branches, which often include libraries with free publications.

Common sense rule: Identify the resources that help you the most and learn from these.

No matter where you get your information—from person, print, or PC—consider your source. It's usually best to start with reliable organizations, such as the NIH, which are not trying to sell something and which have a good scientific and medical foundation. Unethical businesses (Web-based or bricks-and-mortar) may take advantage of the most vulnerable members of society, including the sick and elderly. Remember that the Food and Drug Administration does not routinely regulate herbs, vitamins, minerals, etc., so manufacturers and marketers of these may make just about any claim that they want. This point is so important as to reiterate, these alternate therapies can be marketed on the basis of unproven statements. Check with a doctor and/or other trusted sources—who do not sell such items.

Common sense rule: Caveat caregiver!

What if I Can't Get My Loved One to the Doctor for Memory Problems?

The most common obstacle in getting a loved one with suspected dementia to a doctor for evaluation is his or her lack of insight into memory or similar deficits. A person with dementia may take offense at a suggestion of memory problems (or similar), having to see a new doctor regarding such and/or having a family member come along. Often the less said, the better. The more routine and nonchalant the process is the more likely it is to proceed.

Most patients will listen to their doctor. So, as suggested above, start with the primary care physician. Find out when the patient's next appointment is and accompany him or her to it (without creating a lot of fanfare). If this is out of the norm and the patient questions you about your going along, tell him or her honestly that you have some questions for the doctor. (If your loved one is suspicious or balks at the idea of your presence at their appointment, call the office and/or fax or mail a note advising the doctor of your concerns. Although physicians cannot discuss a patient's care without consent, they can freely accept any pertinent information.)

Most people say they don't like doctors but usually have a good relationship with their personal physician and willingly follow the direction of their personal physicians to see a specialist. If not, you may wish to see if the primary care doctor is comfortable evaluating and treating dementia—or at least making a start (it may be possible to consult with a specialist later).

Sometimes patients are willing to see a specialist for a problem other than a cognitive one. Someone who is unwilling to see a neurologist for memory loss may be willing—or even eager—to do so for problems with pain, insomnia, or problems with gait (walking) or balance. Stigma regarding seeing a psychiatrist may be conquered by explaining that such a doctor is expert in reviewing medications to see if any can cause or contribute to issues with memory, energy level, or sleep. It is okay if a loved one's chief concern is different from yours.

If none of these measures are successful, and you can't even get the patient to see a primary care doctor, consider exploring the option of geriatric house calls. You can check with local hospitals regarding availability. If geriatric house calls are not available in the patient's locale, consider hiring a professional geriatric care manager to perform a home evaluation and assessment of the needs of the patient and family. Call the Alzheimer Association helpline or consult the Website as to other suggestions and resources. Finally, if a patient's basic health and safety are at risk, it may be necessary to get emergency or adult protective services involved. Unfortunately, emergency services and hospitals are not optimal for dealing with a chronic problem like dementia, so families may be back to square one if a patient is discharged home immediately due to lack of medical justification for hospitalization or after a brief hospital stay. Adult protective services may make decisions for the patient independent of family input. Happily, in most cases it doesn't come to this.

Common sense rule: A patient's chief concern/s should be respected and may differ from a caregiver's. The priority is to obtain appropriate medical evaluation.

Summary

As we mentioned in the beginning of this chapter, the major steps involved in getting help are (1) advocating for the person with dementia; (2) identifying a physician/s who can provide appropriate assessment, diagnosis, and plan (and accompanying the patient to visits with said doctor/s); and (3) seeking additional resources for the patient and for the caregiver. The next chapter will expand on these steps and assist any family member to act as a strong patient advocate in acquiring the knowledge and answers you seek as you accompany your loved one to the doctor. Now that you know where to go for help, the next two chapters show you how to get the answers you need.

Common Sense Rules

- Someone with memory problems (or similar) should not go to the doctor alone.
- A good advocate may have to speak out and—know when to say no.
- Everyone should have a primary care physician.
- See the primary medical doctor first.
- Experience and training are more important than title.
- Unusual medical cases deserve the attention of a specialist.
- Caveat caregiver! (Carefully consider the source of any information.)
- A patient's chief concern/s should be respected and may differ from a caregiver's. The priority is to obtain appropriate medical evaluation.

Websites

Alzheimer's Association: www.alz.org
AAGP: www.aagponline.org
Association for Frontotemporal Degeneration: www.theaftd.org
National Association of Professional Geriatric Care Managers: www.caremanager.org
Lewy Body Dementia Assocation: www.lbda.org
NIH/National Institute on Aging: www.nia.nih.gov and www.nia.nih.gov/Alzheimer's

References

1. Finucane TE, Christmas C, Travis K. Tube feeding in patients with advanced dementia: a review of the evidence. JAMA. 1999;282(14):1365–70.
2. Gillick MR. Rethinking the role of tube feeding in patients with advanced dementia. N Engl J Med. 2000;342(3):206–10.
3. Meier DE, Ahronheim JC, Morris J, Baskin-Lyons S, Morrison RS. High short-term mortality in hospitalized patients with advanced dementia: lack of benefit of tube feeding. Arch Intern Med. 2001;161(4):594–9.
4. Teno JM, Mitchell SL, Kuo SK, Gozalo PL, Rhodes RL, Lima JC, Mor V. Decision-making and outcomes of feeding tube insertion: a five-state study. J Am Geriatr Soc. 2011;59:881–6.
5. Wilkins CH, Wilkins KL, Meisel M, Depke M, Williams J, Edwards DF. Dementia undiagnosed in poor older adults with functional impairment. J Am Geriatr Soc. 2007;55(11):1771–6.

Chapter 4
Preparing for a Visit to the Doctor

"Chance favors the prepared mind."

—Louis Pasteur

Chapter 3 explained the who, what, and where of locating a dementia specialist and other resources. Now, we show you how to ensure that the doctor gets the information necessary to assist a patient and family get the help they need.

If you are a family member, this chapter should prepare you and your loved one for the doctor's visit and set the stage to find the answers you seek. Anyone else who plans to accompany the patient to the clinic may also find it useful. Finally, it may be beneficial for professionals in acquiring complete medical records and laying the foundation for a successful medical evaluation for dementia.

We offer a checklist (Table 4.1) to assist you on this mission and will review each component in detail in this chapter. To make the most of a visit with a doctor, do everything you can in advance to maximize the precious—and limited—amount of face-time that you will have.

Common sense rule: Be prepared.

Before You Go to the Doctor

Making an Appointment

Setting up a doctor's visit may seem obvious and routine, but it is a little different when you are arranging an appointment for someone else. We have found a number of tips that facilitate the process—and may get you and your loved one in to see the doctor sooner.

A.M. Lipton and C.D. Marshall, *The Common Sense Guide to Dementia for Clinicians and Caregivers*, DOI 10.1007/978-1-4614-4163-2_4, © Springer Science+Business Media, LLC 2013

Table 4.1 Checklist for doctor's appointment

• Obtain basic demographics (address, etc.), insurance, and pharmacy plan details and make copies of cards/information
• Make appointment with primary care doctor
– Obtain recommendation/referral for specialist
• Make appointment with specialist
• Obtain medical records including neuroimaging compact discs or films and medical Power of Attorney documents
• Medication list including:
– Allergies/sensitivities
– Doctors' names, #'s, and specialties
– Pharmacy name and #
• Medical history summary including patient's past medical and surgical history and family history
• Your list with current symptoms and your questions and concerns
• For a patient in a long-term care facility:
• Notify facility in advance of any doctor's visits
• Request a copy of the Medication Administration Record (MAR) to bring to each doctor's visit
• Request blank order form/note from care facility

Many people delay this step—Don't! Most specialists and dementia centers have a waiting period which may be up to several months long. What this means is that if you delay setting up the appointment for days or weeks or months, you may have to wait not only that long but even a few months more before seeing the doctor. So, call to make an appointment as soon as you have a recommendation and/or doctor's referral, if needed.

If you want to try to get in sooner and your schedule is flexible, ask if the doctor has a waiting list in case of cancelations and ask to be placed on this. (If you do, make sure to have completed all of the necessary paperwork and know how to get to the doctor's office, so that you can be ready quickly in case you are called.)

Common sense rule: The earlier you call, the sooner you will get answers.

Most of the time, a patient's family member will be the one calling a specialist's office to arrange appointments. Have your calendar (as well as the patient's) handy when you call, in order to schedule the date and time that work best for everyone. Be sure that you have a patient's basic demographics (name, date of birth, address, phone number, etc.), contact information for primary and referring physicians, and insurance card/s and information. You should also make sure that the doctor's office has your name and phone number as the contact person. Even though it has always been our office procedure to obtain all of these details, we have still encountered situations in which we have only had the patient's phone number on file and were unable to reach a family caregiver regarding an appointment (e.g., a reminder phone call or schedule change) and an appointment has been forgotten or a chance for an earlier appointment missed. Make sure that the doctor's office also has your name and address so that such items as forms, appointment reminders, and bills will be mailed to you.

Common sense rule: Don't rely on someone with significant memory loss (or similar) to schedule or remember appointments, etc.

The doctor's office may request—or require—medical records from a patient's doctor, doctors, and/or hospitalization/s, as well as any neuroimaging (CT, MRI, and PET scans). Some clinics prefer to handle this on their own as a doctor-to-doctor process. Unfortunately, sometimes requests go unheeded and records aren't sent. They can also be misfiled or somehow otherwise not available. We therefore encourage you to find out exactly what records a doctor needs and hand-carry them with you to the appointment. This acts as a fail-safe if one doctor's office is unable to obtain records from another or can't find ones that were sent. If you want to drop off the records yourself (or the doctor's office requests or requires this), do so only after making copies for yourself. If you request any neuroimaging, get at least one copy of each test and report on a compact disc for yourself (and future reference). You should also bring copies of any medical Power of Attorney documents. Use your favorite type of organizer to keep everything handy, portable, and in one place.

Common sense rule: Make and file copies of medical records.

Some offices, clinics, hospitals, or neuroimaging facilities may charge a patient or patient's family representative or medical POA for records (but don't charge treating physicians for the same). We would prefer that patients and families avoid the burden of such a fee. So, if you run into this problem, make sure that the dementia specialist's office has all the contact information needed to obtain such records and CALL and make sure that they have all of these records as far in advance of the appointment as you can. If the new doctor hasn't received records from any of these sources, request that the staff try again. Most importantly, avail yourself of this opportunity to directly contact the source yourself, explain the situation, and offer to pick up the record … IF it can be provided free of charge! (And, as always try to obtain or make a copy for your files.)

Common sense rule: Provide relevant past medical records to a new doctor.

Most dementia specialists need recent labs and notes from a patient's primary physician (and/or any other doctor who is referring the patient to the specialist). If a patient has seen a psychiatrist or neurologist recently, *for whatever reason*, these records are usually extremely valuable. Of course, the results of any prior dementia evaluation should also be made available. These include any doctor's notes, neuropsychological evaluations, and results of any prior neuroimaging, such as CT, MRI, and PET scans of the brain or head. The specialist will want to read the radiologist's report of the neuroimaging and may also want to review the actual images. Check with your specialist's office as to whether it is best to bring such neuroimaging results in on a compact disc or via printed copies of the films. This can avoid wasted time and unnecessary repetition of tests.

Of course, it's a good idea to make sure you have everything, but we generally find it's best to leave a detailed review of the medical records to the doctor. It may be depressing and/or anxiety-provoking for a patient or family member to read through these as they general focus on problems and abnormalities. In this case, a little knowledge can truly be a dangerous thing. If you are really interested, you might ask the doctor for an overview.

Common sense rule: Bring medical records directly to the doctor.

Forms

We know that medical forms can be time-consuming and seem redundant. And, we all hate to do paperwork. However, this is a necessary and important step. It also allows for a physician to spend less time gathering a medical history and more time to spend with a patient and family in discussing diagnosis and answering questions. So, our recommendation is—just do it!

First, find out if the doctor has any new patient forms and obtain these from the office, by mail, fax, or via an online Website. Complete these in full and find out if you need to mail or fax these to the doctor's office or bring them in at the time of the appointment. You may wish to call ahead of the appointment and verify that all paperwork has been received. Make sure to indicate in a prominent place if you are completing forms for someone else and your relation to them and/or any Medical Power of Attorney. Be certain to make a copy (or copies) for yourself and bring these to the visit.

Common sense rule: Complete all necessary forms and make copies for yourself.

Medication List

One of the most important reasons to see a specialist (or any doctor) is for a review of medications, determining which may help—or harm—memory and other aspects of a patient's health, and adjusting them accordingly. No changes can be made unless a physician knows what a patient is—and is not—taking. New drugs can't be prescribed (due to risk for duplication or adverse drug reactions) and old ones can't be altered without this knowledge. A new cognitive enhancer can't be added and something that might be hurting memory can't be withdrawn.

We can't tell you how many times that we have heard, "I forgot the medication list. Can I call/fax/email it to you later?" A doctor must have an accurate medication list at each appointment to review current medications and make changes (including additions), as appropriate. Having this information after the appointment doesn't allow the doctor, patient, or family member to make the most of this visit. And, no one wants to have to wait until the next visit if there are any problems, issues, or potential new medications that could and/or should be addressed immediately.

Common sense rule: A doctor can't prescribe new medications (or make changes to old ones) without knowing what a patient is already taking.

Thus, a medication list is one of the most important tools that you can bring to the doctor. Here are some helpful hints to ensure that you always have a medication list in hand. Make sure to verify the accuracy of the medication list before each appointment.

We recommend that everyone should keep such a record with them at all times. A patient's spouse and adult children should also have a list of a loved one's medications—whether the patient has dementia or not!—close at hand. It may be recorded on a smart phone or typed or neatly written in ink and carried in a wallet or purse. (We don't recommend lamination as this makes changes difficult to record.) It may be self-evident that always carrying such an inventory may be life-saving in case of a medical emergency, but you might be surprised how often it comes in handy. You may be extremely grateful to rely on having it with you in every doctor's office, at the pharmacy, or on vacation.

Anyone with a mobile phone should designate an ICE (In Case of Emergency) contact, in addition to listing their medications, for emergency personnel. Patients on certain medications, such as blood thinners, should also wear a medical-alert identification band, as this may also provide life-saving information.

Common sense rule: Always carry a list of medications.

The following are some tips on creating such an inventory. If paperwork from the doctor includes a place to record medications, then, by all means, use their preferred format. If not, we are including a sample template form that will help get you started (Table 4.2).

A complete list should include the name of each medication, dosage (how much), frequency (how often), indication (reason for taking medications), and the name of the prescribing doctor. Make sure to be clear about the dosage and frequency. For example, if you say that a pill is taken as "two a day," it is unclear as to whether two pills are taken once daily or one pill is taken twice daily. A doctor needs to know which one is the case, so be as specific as you can. If a pill is taken once daily, indicate at approximately what time or, at least, whether it is taken in the AM, PM, or midday. Note if a pill is taken with food (after a meals or a specific meal) or on an empty stomach (before meals or a specific meal). **Include all over-the-counter medications, vitamins, minerals, herbal remedies, and all other supplements.** All of these have potential risks, benefits, and interactions with each other. We have placed this statement in bold because, even though we included this instruction in our own office medication form, it has often been neglected. We have often had to apply considerable effort to determine whether a patient is taking something perceived to be innocuous (perhaps because it doesn't require a prescription or is an alternative or natural remedy), but which may actually interfere with memory, pose other risks, or interact with other substances.

If a patient self-dispenses medication and uses a list, make sure to bring that, too. If a family member, companion, or professional administer medication, bring the

Table 4.2 Blank medication form

Patient name: _____

ALLERGIES: _____

Emergency contact name and number: _____

MEDICATION LIST

Date that this list was last updated: ____/____/_____ (month/date/year)

Please list all of your medications, including prescription, over-the-counter, vitamins, and herbal supplements

Medication	Dosage (e.g., mg)	Frequency (e.g. AM, PM, twice daily)	Reason for taking	Doctor who prescribes this medication
_____	_____	_____	_____	_____
_____	_____	_____	_____	_____
_____	_____	_____	_____	_____
_____	_____	_____	_____	_____
_____	_____	_____	_____	_____
_____	_____	_____	_____	_____

Pharmacy: _____ Phone: _____

Primary Doctor: _____ Phone: _____

Other Doctor: _____ Phone: _____

list utilized to do so. If your loved one lives in a supervised living community and the staff administer medications, ask for a copy of the patient's Medication Administration Record (MAR) that you can bring to the doctor's office. Do not assume that the facility will automatically send the MAR to the doctor or give it to you without a specific request. Make sure to obtain any such list/s in advance of the appointment and verify for accuracy.

Medication Administration Record

Request a copy of the MAR to bring to every doctor's visit. Although a facility may offer to fax the MAR to your physician's office, your better bet is to bring it with you. Call ahead and let the staff know that you will need it by a certain time. This helps prevent delays when you are rushing to get your loved one out the door in time for an appointment, and you find the staff is away from the desk attending to other patients.

Another reason to obtain this in advance is to ensure that it is up-to-date. Most MARs are printed at the beginning of the month and will have the month and year clearly displayed on the document. Since medication changes can occur throughout the month, each MAR system has a way to address how the changes make it into the document. No need to concern yourself with the details so much as to talk to the nurse and make sure you leave the facility with everything you need.

Most MARs include two basic sections. One section lists the medications, doses, and scheduled administration times. The other section records the actual administrations of the medication. Some facilities send only the medication list and remove the daily administration log. So if you are given strips of paper (essentially they look like scissors were taken to them) versus regular size paper, you can assume the administration portion is absent. It is crucial that the administration portion of the MAR is included so that your physician can monitor each use of medications, particularly those given PRN (as needed).

For example, the administration record may help a reviewing physician determine whether a medication was refused by the patient or held by a nurse due to sedation. The physician might observe that a patient took an antibiotic for a week for a urinary tract infection. Such an infection might cause a delirium and explain why a patient was more confused during that period.

As dementia specialists, we look for patient compliance and use of PRN (as needed) medication.

Without knowing compliance, a doctor might increase a medication dosage, mistakenly assuming that the prescribed amount is not effective, rather than the patient is refusing the medication. If we see that compliance is typically a problem at night, we may move some medication to earlier in the day. If a patient needs PRN agitation or anxiety medications, that gives us a great deal of clinical information and directs the next step of the treatment. For example if a patient needs such medications one or more times daily, consideration may be made to adding a medication to help prevent or better address such agitation or anxiety.

It is important to bring and review the MAR even if you have your own list. In our practice, families may not have brought the current MAR because they are confident "nothing has changed." Remember this is a complex system involving patients, multiple medical providers, family members, and facility staff. And let's not forget the pharmacy—or the hospital, skilled nursing, rehabilitation unit, or other facility, if a patient is admitted or transferred to one of these.

Then consider that within the greater system, individuals communicate via multiple domains: in person; via phone, fax, electronic communication, and/or printed and/or written discharge and other orders; or by sending written orders with patient or family. The chances for miscommunication loom large. By viewing the MAR regularly, physicians can easily verify if treatment plan is being followed. It is also important for families to review. In fact, it is a good idea for a relative to obtain a copy of the MAR (with appropriate consent) and review this for accuracy on a regular basis (at least every few months). It should also be checked after any major transition for the patient, such as a move or hospitalization, to ensure that it has been properly updated. You might be surprised at what you find. We have had family members learn (much to their dismay) that loved ones had received the wrong drug or dosage (or an important medication had been omitted) based on an incorrect or out-of-date MAR. Just because you are aware of changes doesn't guarantee that they have been implemented. And, even if you have not been made aware of any changes, doesn't mean that none have occurred.

Common sense rule: If a patient has a Medication Administration Record (MAR), review it and bring it to every doctor's visit.

Medication Bottles and Pillboxes

We find a list serves as the quickest and most effective way of learning about a patient's medications. However, some doctors prefer to have the bottles of medication brought into the office. If you're not sure, err on the side of caution and do both (make a list and bring in the bottles). In some cases, especially for over-the-counter remedies containing multiple components, a doctor may need to review the label for the complete listing of ingredients. The label and contents of the bottle may also aid in determining whether a patient is taking a medication as prescribed (e.g., if a medication should be taken daily and was filled more than 90 days ago with 90 pills and pills still remain). Therefore, whenever possible, bring medication bottles with labels as well as a list. (We highly recommend the use of pillboxes, but having pillboxes alone doesn't provide the all-important labeling information and makes medication identification more challenging and time-consuming.)

Medication Allergies and Sensitivities

Include any medication allergies and sensitivities along with a list of current medications. List not only the medication but also the specific problem associated with it.

All medication allergies are sensitivities, but not all medication sensitivities are true allergies. Specific symptoms are associated with an allergic reaction. These include rash, shortness of breath/swelling of the mouth and/or throat (anaphylaxis), and/or low blood pressure (hypotension or shock).

A medication sensitivity, on the other hand, may relate to any adverse effect/s associated with a particular drug for a given individual. It could be associated with almost any symptom, such as nausea, vomiting, or dizziness. For example, nausea and vomiting are known adverse effects of codeine. Some people experience these effects with this drug and some do not. Someone who has nausea and vomiting (but no other symptoms) while taking codeine may have a sensitivity to this medication but isn't experiencing a true allergic reaction.

It's best to list all medication allergies and sensitivities by identifying each drug and problem it has caused in the past as specifically as possible (e.g., penicillin caused a rash on the chest and back, codeine caused nausea and vomiting). This will help a doctor determine what medications should be avoided and which might be tried again with caution, if needed. Medical-alert identification bands may be life-saving for patients with known allergies to medications or other triggers. And, doctors and other medical personnel also need to know about these other types of allergies/triggers to allergic reactions, such as food allergies, bee stings, etc.

Common sense rule: Carry a list of specific medication allergies/sensitivities.

Pharmacy, Prescriber, and Prescription Information

Pharmacy and doctor information also belongs on a medication list. If you don't have room, then you should keep this information in your mobile phone or make another list. Include pharmacy name and number as well as doctors' names, specialties, phone numbers, and fax numbers, if possible.

Bring the patient's prescription plan card and information to every doctor's appointment. Be familiar with a patient's prescription plan and what it covers, especially regarding any cost savings regarding the number of days' supply of medication or mail order. Some plans offer discounts for bulk orders (e.g., 90 days' supply rather than filling a 30-day supply thrice) and/or ordering by mail. A doctor will need to know if he or she should write for a 30- or 90-day supply of medication, and if the prescriptions will be filled locally or by mail order.

For Patients in Supervised Care Facilities

It is best to advise long-term care facility of doctors' visits ahead of time. In addition to providing you with the MAR (see above), you may also request a blank order form and a blank progress note, so that the physician can effectively communicate any new orders and instructions.

History

When listing the history, think like a doctor and make a brief list of a patient's medical history. Key highlights are much more important than noting details. Use a doctor's own form, if available. If not, this history should not be more than one page. Include any injury a patient has had that may be relevant to a dementia evaluation, particularly head injury and/or loss of consciousness (blacking out). For the patient and family, make sure to include diseases that may impinge upon a dementia diagnosis, such as strokes. Make sure to include any history of dementia in the family with age and symptoms of onset, if known. This inventory should include:

Medical history: Any significant injuries and illness, including date of onset, if known.

Surgical history: Any significant surgeries, including year performed, if known. For more recent procedures, it may be helpful to list the month or exact date, if known.

Family history:

Number of all of a patient's biological siblings or half-siblings. Include current ages, if living, or age and cause of death, if deceased. List whether they have memory problems or not.

Significant diseases in biological relatives (those related by blood, rather than marriage or adoption), including parents, siblings, and children (We have found that many adult children of our patients don't think to include their own medical history, so we remind you to do so, when relevant.) If any of these close relatives has died, include age of death and cause of death.

Family neurological/psychiatric history: Include any history of neurological and psychiatric illness and hospitalizations, such as strokes, Parkinson's disease or similar, amyotrophic lateral sclerosis (ALS, also called Lou Gehrig's disease), depression, alcoholism, bipolar disorder, etc.

Family dementia history (Since this is directly relevant, it can be a bit more detailed and include whatever information is known. Age of onset, symptoms, and diagnosis, if any are particularly helpful.): Include any history of dementia or memory problems in a patient's biological aunts and uncles as well as the close relatives listed above.

Social history: If you are feeling particularly ambitious, you can also prepare this. A social history typically takes account of any past or present history of alcohol, tobacco, or other substances. For a dementia evaluation, it is crucial to know a patient's education, present or former occupation (specify whether the patient working or retired), and living situation (e.g., lives alone at home or with a spouse in a senior living apartment). You can also add any hobbies or exercise.

Common sense rule: Make sure the doctor is aware of any relevant patient and family medical history.

Table 4.3 shows a sample history:

Your List

We saved the best for last. This list is for you. If you do nothing else, do this—for yourself, your loved one, and the doctor.

Type (or neatly write) your top 1–3 concerns/questions. Always start with the worst, most pressing problem first. Highlight each with a word or few words (e.g., memory loss, agitation, aggression, hallucinations), so that it's easy to see what the problem is. You can then add a line, few lines, or paragraph with one or more examples. It should be no longer than a page, or you are including too much detail. Summarize overall features by theme (rather than listing specific examples), if you need to make it shorter. A day-to-day diary documenting day-by-day events and behavior is not particularly helpful as it doesn't easily allow a doctor to discern a pattern. Remember the ABCs of dementia and emphasize key problems with Activities of Daily Living, Behavior, and Cognition (thinking/mental processes).

Include in your note the key points that the physician needs to know about such symptoms, including onset (when the problem started), frequency (how often it occurs), timing (when it occurs, e.g., more often in the evening), and any known

Table 4.3 Sample patient history prepared by family member for doctor

Patient Name: Jane Smith

Date of Birth: 1/1/1938

Past Medical History

Breast cancer, in remission. Diagnosed age 72. Had chemotherapy and mastectomy

Strokes seen by doctor on CAT scan but no history of any stroke symptoms

High blood pressure (diagnosed in her 40s)

High cholesterol (diagnosed in her 60s)

Hypothyroidism (diagnosed in her 50s)

3 pregnancies, 1 miscarriage and 2 live births (1 C-section)

Past Surgical History

Appendectomy in her 20s

Mastectomy January 2011 (age 73)

Family History

Oldest of four children.

    1 brother died of a heart attack in his 60s.

    Patient's two living sisters have high blood pressure and 1 had a stroke in her 60s, but neither
        has memory problems.

Father died in his 40s in a car accident

Mother died of a stroke age 81 in a nursing home and had memory problems for the last 5 years
    of her life that became progressively worse. She never had a diagnosis for this by a doctor,
    but the family thinks she had Alzheimer's disease. None of mother's 6 siblings (patient's
    maternal aunts and uncles) or any of patient's other relatives are known to have had any
    memory problems. Besides strokes and possible dementia, there is no family history of
    neurological or psychiatric illness

Both grown children have high blood pressure

Social History

Married, lives at home with husband John

Graduated from the state university and worked as an office manager for 40+ years. Retired age 62

2 adult children, Audrey and Bill

Never smoked

Drinks 1 glass of wine with dinner

Hobbies/exercise: Reading, cooking, bridge. Walks 1 mile daily

---

triggers (e.g., being in a strange environment like a hotel or hospital). Don't obscure major problems with too much information. A little really does go a long way—and is often better. Usually, just one or two examples can make your point. Give one copy to the doctor and bring a copy for yourself as well as a pen and pad of paper so that you can take notes on the answers.

Common sense rule: Prioritize problems and deal with the worst first.

Here is a sample note (Table 4.4):

Table 4.4 Sample note from family member for doctor

Dear Doctor:

These are my major concerns for my dad and why I am bringing him to see you today. As his daughter (and the only one of his family who lives locally), I'd like to know any medical cause for these problems and the best ways for me to help him handle these problems:

1. Memory loss.

   This is Dad's worst problem and the main reason for our visit. He began having minor memory problems about 2 years ago and they have gotten worse since then. He now forgets conversations after a few minutes and sometimes calls me back on the phone right after we have just spoken. He has also occasionally forgotten to take his daily medication

2. Problems managing finances.

   I found out that Dad got a late bill notice which is very unusual for him. I then sat down with him and we looked at his finances together. I noticed that he had actually paid some of his bills twice

3. Driving.

   Dad had to call me for directions to the bank he has been using for many years and becomes upset when reminded of this.

Sensitive Subjects

Some problems are understandably difficult to discuss in front of the person experiencing them. These may include driving, finances, alcohol consumption, urinary or bowel incontinence (wetting or soiling oneself), physical and/or verbal aggression, hallucinations (usually seeing or hearing things in the case of dementia), and paranoid delusions, including delusions of marital infidelity (a person mistakenly believes that their spouse is being unfaithful).

We don't want you to ever have to make a phone call to a doctor like this: I was with my mother at her appointment with you this morning. I am calling to give you more information because there was a lot that I was not comfortable discussing in front of her.

We certainly understand a family member's hesitation in bringing up sensitive information in the presence of a patient. Families worry that the information will be upsetting to their loved one. Or that the patient will deny it and an argument will erupt. Rest assured that physicians experienced in dementia can handle these sensitive topics during an appointment. However, the doctor needs to know everything at that time in order to address these issues. Calling with pertinent information after the visit is disruptive and makes the whole process inefficient. Often, the doctor will have begun implementation of a treatment plan, including medication recommendations, and discussed that with you and the patient, on the basis of the information gathered at the appointment. Knowing the full picture is vital not only in the approach to the problem, including what drugs to prescribe, but also in making a diagnosis.

One helpful suggestion is to include these topics in your note, indicating what subjects have or may be particularly distressing to the patient (see Table 4.4 for an example), and deliver it discreetly to the doctor. You can do this via a variety of means. You might enclose it in an envelope addressed to the doctor and hand it to office staff during check-in to pass on to the doctor. You could also fax or email it the day before or morning of an appointment. You may wish to call the clinic and ensure that it has been received.

If you need to discuss these issues further, you might inquire as to whether you could schedule a family conference with the doctor—and without the patient. Some doctors may offer this type of visit, provided appropriate consent for release of patient information has been obtained. Make sure to check regarding any charge associated with such an appointment. Unfortunately, insurance may not cover costs for any visits without the patient present. You can circumspectly inquire about such a meeting in your note to the doctor, a quiet word to the front desk, or a call to the office.

Common sense rule: Communicate your concerns effectively in order to have them fully understood and addressed.

Summary

Before you go to the doctor's office, prepare in advance. Call early for an appointment. Collect records and summarize a patient's medical history. Compose a list of medications. Make a note of your concerns for yourself and the doctor.

Common Sense Rules

- The earlier you call, the sooner you will get answers.
- Don't rely on someone with significant memory loss (or similar) to remember appointments, etc.
- Make and file copies of medical records.
- Provide relevant past medical records to a new doctor.
- Always carry a list of medications.
- If a patient has a Medication Administration Record (MAR), review it and bring it to every doctor's visit.
- Make sure the doctor is aware of any relevant patient and family medical history.
- Prioritize problems and deal with the worst first.
- Communicate your concerns effectively in order to have them fully understood and addressed.

Chapter 5
Making the Most of the Doctor's Visit

"First do no harm."

—Hippocrates

"Second, do some good."

— Anne M. Lipton, M.D., Ph.D.

Every patient and family has a story. In this chapter, we present some effective ways of sharing yours. The last chapter prepared you for the doctor's visit. Here, we help you make the most of it once you've arrived. And, being there is essential. Someone with memory loss (or similar problems) should have someone responsible with them to act as a patient advocate. Otherwise, the physician may not receive an accurate history (upon which the correct diagnosis depends) or the patient may forget essential matters, such as medication instructions.

This chapter offers important insights into the ways in which a physician thinks— specifically, the methods by which a doctor obtains medical details and organizes these facts to facilitate pattern-recognition and reach a diagnosis. We remind you of the materials that you should bring along, help you determine what questions you should be sure to ask, and share tried-and-true tips to enable you to successfully communicate your concerns—and, most important of all, to elicit answers.

Anyone accompanying a patient to a medical office or otherwise acting as a patient advocate may find this information valuable. It should enhance the clarity of communication and the free-flowing exchange of ideas and information among all involved in the interaction. This includes doctors, who may find it helpful as a reminder that their process is not always intuitive, and that they should take care to provide straightforward explanations to nonphysicians.

A patient and family should work together with the doctor towards the best medical management of dementia via the following steps: (1) Identification of the problem or problems; (2) Communication of these issues and other medical history to the physician; (3) Dementia evaluation including physical examination, neuroimaging, and laboratory tests; (4) Finding out the results of all evaluations performed as well as a specific diagnosis; and (5) Formulation of a plan of treatment.

A.M. Lipton and C.D. Marshall, *The Common Sense Guide to Dementia for Clinicians and Caregivers*, DOI 10.1007/978-1-4614-4163-2_5, © Springer Science+Business Media, LLC 2013

Common sense rule: Someone with memory issues (or similar problems) should not go alone to doctor's visits.

What You Need to Bring to the Doctor's Office

In this case, it's really "who" rather than "what." Someone who knows the patient well should plan to attend the doctor's appointment (and that means not just dropping a patient off or waiting for him or her in the waiting room, but being mentally, physically, and emotionally prepared and present throughout the visit). Ideally, a family member who lives with the patient and/or will be involved in the patient's care on an ongoing basis should attend. So, if that's you, the most important thing to bring is yourself.

The following encounter illustrates a common problem that can and should be avoided:

> A 76 year-old woman with Alzheimer's disease and her adult son attend a follow-up visit with a dementia specialist. The patient had been having insomnia and the doctor prescribed a medication to help with this. When the doctor asked about her current quality of sleep, the patient was unable to recall if she was still having problems. Her adult son added, "I'm sorry, but I really don't know if Mom is sleeping better. Mom lives with my sister, but I am trying to help more. One way to help was to bring Mom to her appointment today."

We completely understand that patients' families are busy and have conflicts with appointments. We fully support family caregivers taking care of themselves by attending to work and other commitments. That being said, we recommend that a family member who knows the patient well attend all physician visits. If that is not possible, assign one family member to a particular doctor. This helps with consistency and communication. After each appointment, that relative can email or otherwise communicate the pertinent findings and treatment recommendations to other family members. You could then bring a printed email or notes on the information with you to your assigned physician. If family cannot attend in person, ask if your physician's office has an option to include you on speaker phone during the appointment. If all of a patient's relatives live out-of-town, consider hiring a geriatric care manager to accompany your loved one to appointments and communicate the findings with family.

We welcome all relatives to be involved in the care of a family member with dementia, but someone should be designated as the point person. Ideally, this individual should live with (or close) to the patient, interact with the patient on a routine basis, and maintain a record of patient's basic medical history, current symptoms, and any medications or allergies (see Chap. 4). Such coordination and consistency optimizes a patient's overall care. Without such a system in place, a family and/or doctor may lack awareness of or the means to address key medical issues.

Common sense rule: A patient with dementia should have a medical advocate.

Table 5.1 Checklist of items to bring to the doctor's visit

- Patient's photo ID
- Insurance and pharmacy plan cards
- Medical records, including neuroimaging reports (images on films or CD if requested)
- Medical power of attorney documents
- Medication list including:
  - Allergies/sensitivities
  - Doctors' names, #'s, and specialties
  - Pharmacy name and #
- Medical history summary including patient's past medical and surgical history and family history
- Your list with current symptoms and your questions and concerns
- Any assistive device, including eyeglasses, hearing aids, dentures, cane, walker, wheelchair, or similar

For a patient in long-term care facility:

- Notify facility in advance of any doctor's visits
- Request a copy of the Medication administration record (MAR) to bring to each doctor's visit
- Request blank order form/note from care facility

Bring a pen and pad so you can take notes on the answers

Table 5.1 provides a handy summary of the notes and materials that you need to bring to the appointment (See Chap. 4 for specific details.)

Assistive Devices

Bring any eyeglasses, hearing aids, walkers, canes, or other assistive devices that the patient uses in daily life to facilitate adequate evaluation. If a patient does not have proper visual correction, this may not only impair examination of visual acuity but also of other functions, including reading and writing. If a patient doesn't wear his or her hearing aids or dentures, it may be impossible to adequately test language functions. Leaving a walker or cane at home may preclude assessment of a patient's gait (walking) and balance.

Common sense rule: Bring all of the patient's assistive devices to any medical evaluation.

Communicating with the Doctor

During our clinical interview with a patient and family, we generally elicit and record this primary symptom first from the patient and then from the accompanying family member. It is often very telling to hear the patient's reason for seeking consultation. Sometimes we have written information from the new patient form (which may have been completed by the family) or other records indicating memory loss, and the patient doesn't mention this. In such a case, we mention that we often evaluate people for memory difficulties and specifically ask the patient as to whether he or she is experiencing such problems. We also ask the patient his or her age. This line of questioning can be extremely valuable for a clinicians as it often quickly reveals if a patient has severe deficits of memory and/or insight and whether it may be difficult (or impossible) to obtain an accurate history from the patient:

> An 80 year-old man presented with his daughter for evaluation. The new patient form (completed by the daughter) listed "memory loss" as the chief concern. When asked the reason for his visit to the clinic, the patient replied, "My knees hurt." When asked whether he had any problems with his memory, he demurred, declaring, "no more than anyone else my age." When asked his age, he replied that he didn't know and exhibited a "positive head-tilt," turning towards his daughter as if looking to her for the answer.

Dementia specialists are well aware that patients with advancing dementia may report things incorrectly. Patients with dementia may not have full awareness of memory loss and similar symptoms. Patients in early stages of dementia may have partial insight into their problems, but lack full insight.

Therefore, whereas a family may clearly see memory loss (or another cognitive or behavioral problem) as the main reason for a visit with a dementia specialist, a patient with dementia may or may not. Or, a patient may be able to state a symptom such as memory loss as the chief concern, but is unable to provide full details. Therefore, it is imperative for a family member who can do so to be present at the doctor's visit, but to let the patient speak first and only step in as directed by the physician.

Whenever possible (and not just in a clinic setting), it is best to avoid correcting or arguing with a patient who has dementia. Such efforts are often futile and may be upsetting (and not just to the patient!) or even counterproductive. Many other and better means can guarantee that the doctor has the correct information. Correcting a patient throughout the appointment merely serves to frustrate everyone as exemplified by the exasperated comments of a patient's grown daughter:

> No, Dad, you retired 4 years ago. And you know you aren't sleeping well. You tell me that almost every day. What do you mean you eat well? You eat like a bird.

Common sense rule: Avoid conflict and employ alternate strategies.

Since it can distress a patient for a doctor and family member to discuss these matters (either in front of the patient or not), we strongly recommend that you type or write a brief letter for the doctor listing your major concerns (see Chap. 4, Table 4.3) and hand-carry two copies to the appointment (one copy for the doctor and one for yourself). If a patient is particularly sensitive, you may wish to place the note in an envelope and hand it to the front desk to pass along to the physician. You could also fax it the day before the visit.

Putting it in writing is the best way to assure that you convey essential—and accurate—information, to the doctor.

If you bring a pen and pad of paper to take notes, then you also have the option to write something down for the physician during the visit, if it becomes relevant:

> The grown daughter of a 76 year-old man brought her father for an initial dementia evaluation. The dementia specialist inquired about alcohol use and the patient stated that he drank "two glasses of whiskey daily" but was unable to further quantify the amount. His daughter was taking notes during the interview and handed the doctor a brief one-sentence note to the doctor indicating that the patient was actually drinking a full bottle of whiskey daily.

Common sense rule: Put it in writing.

Other Strategies for Communicating with the Doctor

If space allows, you might also try to position yourself in the office such that you are facing the physician but next to or slightly behind Dad. When Dad asserts he's still working, instead of correcting him, just nod "no." If Dad denies napping, and you observe him sleeping throughout the day, you can nod a "yes." Hearing deficits in your loved one can also used to your advantage as you can whisper the correct answer to the physician.

Most dementia specialists will be able to address a family's concerns with a minimum amount of disruption to the patient, either by a nonchalant discussion or writing down instructions for relatives. If there are additional matters that you wish to discuss further, another option may be to schedule a family visit without the patient (with appropriate consent):

> The adult granddaughter of an 82 year-old woman who lived alone accompanied her grandmother to an initial visit with a dementia specialist. The patient denied any problems but had moderate-to-severe impairments of memory, abstract reasoning, judgment, and visuospatial skills on examination. The granddaughter was reluctant to discuss any issues in front of her grandmother. The patient had consented for her private health information to be discussed with the granddaughter and the patient's grown daughter, and a family visit with both of them and without the patient was scheduled at the doctor's recommendation. Numerous issues were discussed and clarified, including that the patient had been having gradually progressive memory loss for 4 years. Two years before the visit, she stopped driving at her family's behest and they began managing her finances as she was no longer able to keep up with payment of her bills. Over the prior 6 months, she didn't seem to be bathing regularly, wasn't eating well (and was losing weight), and wasn't taking medications as prescribed. In the month or two prior to her visit, she also appeared to have had one or two paranoid delusions that a pizza delivery man was stealing from her despite a lack of evidence. She was diagnosed and treated for Alzheimer's disease. Her family moved her into assisted living where she did well. She enjoyed participating in many of the social and other available activities. Her appetite improved and she returned to her usual weight. She also experienced no further delusions or psychosis over the next few years.

As illustrated above, this type of family meeting (without a patient) may be extremely beneficial. However, not all doctors offer them and most insurance companies won't pay for them, so check to see if it is a possibility and, if so, what the charge will be. Most physicians will not schedule such a visit without first establishing a relationship with a patient, meaning that such a family visit usually can't be held until after an initial evaluation at least. Appropriate patient consent for such a visit must be obtained. If you have questions about this, check with the doctor's office.

How the Doctor's Visit Works

You don't have to talk like a doctor—but, it can't hurt, and it might help. So, here's your crash course in Medicalese 101 and the steps that a physician takes in reaching a diagnosis and plan of care.

History

Chief Concern

Most doctors are taught in medical school to record the patient's main reason for a hospital or clinic visit as the "Chief Complaint." This is not meant to imply that patients are "complainers," but it can sound pejorative. Therefore, we prefer the term "Chief Concern."

It's best to provide the main symptom to be evaluated in a word or short phrase, such as "memory loss," "agitation," or "hallucinations." However, you should be aware of and able to supply further details and specific examples, if requested.

Common sense rule: Always start with the worst, most pressing problem first.

History of Present Illness

A physician collects the details of the Chief Concern (or Concerns) in the History of present illness, or HPI. They include exact symptoms and examples, onset (when and how quickly the symptoms started), frequency (how often does a symptom occur (e.g., Does a patient have hallucinations every night or once a week), duration (how long the symptoms have been going on or how long they last when they occur, contributing factors (anything that makes the symptom/s better or worse), and associated symptoms (e.g., a patient may have started having problems with naming objects for a couple of years but started having falls over the past 6 months). The diagnosis of dementia is a clinical one. Dementia is a terminal illness, which means that different dementias all progress to the same endpoint and are most distinctive early in the course of the illness. In other words, the history of a dementia, particularly the first and worst symptoms, may be key to identification. Therefore, a dementia specialist relies on an accurate HPI to supply the most specific diagnosis.

The "ABCs" of dementia help categorize important primary and/or associated symptoms and can be useful in organizing examples of problems that you wish to share with the doctor:

Activities of Daily Living

Functioning can be divided into Instrumental and Basic Activities of Daily Living (ADLs). Patients with dementia usually have problems with Instrumental ADLs (IADLs) first. This is because these are more complex functions, such as cooking, shopping, managing finances, and driving. Basic ADLs (BADLs) are the fundamentals of day-to-day existence, such as eating, dressing, bathing, and toileting. It is vital for a doctor to know of any problems that may pose a risk to the health, safety, and well-being of a patient—and/or others (such as an individual who persists in driving despite an inability to operate a vehicle safely).

Behavior

Make sure to let the doctor know about any significant changes in the patient's mood, behavior, or personality. Examples of mood symptoms might include agitation, apathy, depression, euphoria, and/or irritability. Behavioral changes might include aggression (verbal, physical, and/or sexual), disinhibition (saying and doing inappropriate things), and psychosis. When a patient experiences psychosis, he or she "loses touch" with reality in some way. Psychosis may include hallucinations and/or delusions. A hallucination is an imagined sensory experience (e.g., seeing, hearing, or feeling something that isn't really there). The most common hallucinations in dementia are visual ("seeing things") or auditory ("hearing things"). A delusion is a false belief or mistaken idea (e.g., patient mistakenly believes family member is an imposter, stealing, or having an affair).

Be sure to make the doctor aware of some examples as well as how often these symptoms occur and how troubling they are to you and the patient. This information may be critical to the doctor in making the dementia diagnosis and determining treatment. For example, a patient who had hallucinations once in the hospital after surgery and while on pain medications might not need to be put on a medication for these symptoms, but severe psychosis once or more daily might warrant pharmacologic treatment.

Include any problems with eating, sleeping, or motor behavior. Pacing would be an example of motor behavior. Issues with these behaviors can adversely impact quality of life not only for the patient but also for anyone who lives with them (see Chaps. 11 and 12 for additional information on mood, behavior, and psychosis).

Cognition

Cognitive domains include attention and concentration, memory, language, visuospatial skills (which include hand–eye coordination), and complex thought processes known as executive functions. Memory is the most common first symptom of Alzheimer's disease and many other types of dementia. Let the doctor know what types of things the patient is having difficulty remembering, such as recent events, appointments, conversations, and names. You should provide a couple examples, especially if you can remember the first and/or worst incident/s of forgetting.

If another cognitive domain, such as language, is predominantly affected first, a non-Alzheimer's dementia may be a diagnostic consideration. Non-Alzheimer dementias may also be heralded by noncognitive symptoms, such as problems with gait, strength, or behavior. Therefore, informing a physician of early symptoms may help in making the correct diagnosis.

You can think of the frontal lobes as the Chief Executive Officer (CEO) of the brain. They help coordinate the higher order cognitive processes, known as frontal or executive functions. These include sustained attention, planning, organization, judgment, anticipation, the ability to alternate between tasks (mental set-shifting), and response inhibition (ability to suppress actions). The frontal lobes also mediate emotional states. Patients with frontal lobe damage due to brain injury and/or dementia may therefore exhibit one or more of the following: Apathy/emotional blunting, depression, euphoria, disinhibition, compulsions, and/or perseverative (repetitive) thinking. Patients who are disinhibited may speak or act inappropriately and display a loss of social graces. This could include diverse behaviors but some examples include loudly insulting others, discussing private matters with strangers, or disrobing in public.

Other Medical History

Other elements of the history: Past Medical and Surgical History, Family Medical History, and Social History, and Medications/Allergies/Sensitivities are covered in Chap. 4.

Examination

An evaluation for dementia includes assessing cognitive domains via a mental status, cognitive, neurocognitive, and/or neuropsychological evaluation. Such testing may be performed by a physician or neuropsychologist. A caregiver interview and/ or questionnaire may be included. A physical examination, including a neurological examination, may also be important. While "symptoms" are elicited in the history, a doctor looks for "signs" on examination that may be a clue to diagnosis and/or require further evaluation or treatment. Memory loss is a symptom, but a loss of reflexes is a physical "sign" (and generally not something that most patients or family would be aware of without a physical examination). Like symptoms, signs may help guide diagnosis.

If you are accompanying the patient and wish to be present during any examination, just ask the doctor. Most dementia specialists are happy to include supportive family members whenever possible. Please be cognizant, however, that some testing may need to be done with the patient alone (or the caregiver alone), and the evaluator will let you know.

Additional Evaluation

This may include neuroimaging (such as CT, MRI, PET, or SPECT scans) and laboratory testing. Blood tests are commonly checked as part of an initial dementia evaluation. A spinal tap (lumbar puncture) and/or urine tests may be done in some cases. A detailed explanation of a medical work-up for dementia is beyond the scope of this book but is easily referenced elsewhere [1, 2].

The most important job of a caregiver is not just to make sure these tests are done, but to make know why each is done (and how it might make a difference for the patient), and most importantly, to make sure to find out the results (and get a copy). If the results are somewhat detailed or complicated, such as is often the case for neuroimaging, ask the doctor to go over these with you.

Don't try to memorize all the results. Write down the doctor's explanation. Get copies. If you don't understand anything, especially the meaning and spelling of medical terms—ASK. There's a reason doctors take a lot of notes. Even someone with a normal memory can't be expected to remember everything.

Common sense rule: Get copies of medical test result.

Assessment

A doctor synthesizes the patient history, examination, and results of any other evaluations in deciding on a diagnosis. This is called the assessment. A dementia assessment is complex and involves consideration of many diagnostic possibilities (the "differential diagnosis"). This may include various types of dementia and other possible medical etiologies of symptoms and other findings.

Dementia is considered to be a "clinical diagnosis" in that there is no one test that can be done to diagnose it during life. An accurate dementia diagnosis is therefore highly dependent on the quality of the history provided, the clinical evaluation, and the skill and expertise of the clinician. That is why a thorough evaluation by an experienced dementia specialist may be imperative for proper diagnosis.

Before you leave the doctor's appointment, make sure that you know and understand the diagnosis; the prognosis, including expected duration (if it's a dementia, the prognosis is usually for gradually worsening over years); and the plan of care, which we cover in the next section.

Common sense rule: Ask questions and take notes on test results and diagnosis.

Plan of Care

Newton's Third Law states that for every action, there is an equal and opposite reaction. In medical terms, each clinical assessment or diagnosis deserves a plan of care. And, generally speaking, the more complicated the clinical situation, the more complex the strategy. This is certainly true of dementia which requires a multimodal caregiving approach. This requires much more effort than just taking a pill, although that may be one part of the strategy.

It is important to understand each medication before you leave the doctor's office and have answers to the following questions:

Why (for what reason) is the medication being taken and what benefits are expected?

What are potential side effects?

Is there a generic that can safely be substituted? (Make sure to tell the doctor if cost is an issue.)

Are there any other options (such as alternate medications)?

How is it started? (Titration schedule)

Should any other medications be stopped?

When (what time of day) should it be taken?

Should it be taken with or without food?

In addition to medications, you should consult with the doctor about any treatments other than medication that should be implemented, as well as other sources of help. Non-pharmacologic treatment includes behavioral and environmental measures that may help improve quality of life for the patient and others interacting with the patient. Again, make sure that you understand the reason, method, and expected results of these measures. Find out what professional organization or organizations may help. Ask the physician to provide you with any relevant educational materials available at the clinic.

You should obtain (or make sure the doctor sends) any prescriptions, as well as any referrals for other tests, doctors, or services. These might include physical and/ or occupational therapy (PT/OT), speech-language pathology, home health, or counseling.

Home health services may include nursing care, PT/OT (with possible home safety evaluation) and social work assistance. A patient must meet certain requirements for these services to be covered by insurance, including that the patient doesn't drive. If you're not sure whether your loved one meets the criteria, just ask the doctor if home health might be an option. If a patient qualifies, make sure to request a PT/OT home safety evaluation as this can be an important preventive health measure and may allow insurance coverage of necessary equipment, such as bathtub safety bars, and raised commode seat.

Common sense rule: Make sure you know and understand the plan of care before you leave the doctor's office.

Between Patient Appointments

Keep a symptom log. This needn't be a daily diary, but even just a note in a calendar of an unusual symptom or behavior (as well as the timing—day or night—and any triggers). This should help the doctor identify new problems or patterns, such as worsening insomnia or psychosis.

Know When to Call

Sudden changes demand immediate medical attention (calling 911 for emergency medical assistance). These may include:

- Sudden confusion or change in memory or mood.
- Passing out/serious fall.
- Suddenly unable to speak.
- Sudden weakness.

Inform all of the patient's doctors of any visit to the Emergency Department and/or hospitalization as soon as possible. Call the primary doctor and/or the specialist for any other significant new problems that arise, especially right after starting a new medication (as these may be side effects). Inform the specialist of any new or worsening behavioral issues, such as insomnia, hallucinations, or agitation. Any of these can affect quality of life not only for the patient but also for the caregiver.

Follow-Up on the Plan of Care

Do what you can to follow-up on the plan of care and enlist the help of family, friends, and professionals, where needed. Get additional support from local and national organizations designed to help patients and caregivers. Look for local caregiver courses and symposia. We recommend that all those who will be involved in a patient's care attend a caregiver class at least once. Also educate yourself in other ways that work best for you, whether reading a book like this one or finding resources on the internet. Join a support group, especially if you're feeling isolated.

Talk to your own doctor and ensure that all of your medical problems are optimally treated. Specifically express any changes in your mood, appetite, or sleep. Caregivers may need to see a specialist, too. Consider seeing a counselor if you are anxious, depressed, overwhelmed, or experiencing significant conflict—whether internally or with the patient. A primary care doctor can diagnose depression and prescribe antidepressants, but this is not usually their area of focus. A psychiatrist, especially a geriatric psychiatrist, will be more familiar with the medications and issues faced by caregivers. Such a doctor can also perform psychotherapy or recommend a therapist. A psychiatrist is usually familiar with local counselors who specialize in caregiver therapy. If you aren't getting the answers you need from your physician, you might inquire with your loved one's specialist, a professional association, or fellow caregivers.

Follow-Up Appointments

The doctor who is treating the patient's dementia usually has some specific questions in mind. Make sure to bring yours along as well. Again, it's best to put these in writing for the physician and bring it along with any patient log (as described above), if you've been keeping one.

Your follow-up letter to the doctor should emphasize any changes since the initial visit as well as the effects, if any, of treatment. Make sure to let the doctor know how you're doing, too. Such a note might include:

- The general state of the patient (and caregiver's!) health and well-being.
- Changes (for better or worse) in patient's ADLs, behaviors, and cognition.
- Whether treatments/interventions seem to be working or not.
- Any possible side effects of medication.
- Any new problems (including other aspects of the patient's health or hospital visits).
- A request for any refills needed with the amount needed (such as a 30- or 90-day supply). Also note whether the Rx should be written and given at the visit or sent (and, if it is to be sent, specify which pharmacy).
- Any other requests, questions, or concerns.

At the follow-up visit, again make sure that you understand any new plan of care, including the indication (reason for taking), benefits, and risks of all medications. Obtain (or make sure the doctor sends) any prescriptions, as well as any referrals for other tests, doctors, or services.

Common sense rule: Put it in writing—again!

Summary

Advance preparation and organization can help you make the most of a doctor's visit. Present and highlight important medical information in a structured fashion. Bring and take notes and relevant records. Familiarize yourself with a loved one's medications and prescription needs. Convey your concerns and have them addressed in ways that avoid turmoil. Know what questions to ask — and ask them! Document answers and gather materials that will assist you in caring for your loved one, including finding other means of help to assist you. A well thought-out plan of action is most likely to result in an optimal plan of care. Go home happy knowing what to expect and what to do.

Common Sense Rules

- Someone with memory issues (or similar problems) should not go alone to doctor's visits.
- A patient with dementia should have a medical advocate.
- Bring all of the patient's assistive devices to any medical evaluation.
- Avoid conflict and employ alternate strategies.
- Put it in writing.
- Always start with the worst, most pressing problem first.
- Get copies of medical test result.
- Ask questions and take notes on test results and diagnosis.
- Make sure you know and understand the plan of care before you leave the doctor's office.

References

1. Lipton AM, Rubin CD. Medical evaluation and diagnosis. In: Weiner MF, Lipton AM, editors. The American Psychiatric Publishing Textbook of Alzheimer disease and Other Dementias. Washington, D.C.: American Psychiatric Publishing, Inc.; 2009.
2. Knopman DS, DeKosky ST, Cummings JL, et al. Practice parameter: diagnosis of dementia (an evidence-based review). Report of the Quality Standards Subcommittee of the American Academy of Neurology. Neurology. 2001;56:1143–53.

Part II
Common Sense Dementia Care

Chapter 6
The Seven Common Senses of Dementia Care

Many seeming faults are to be imputed rather to the nature of
the undertaking, than the negligence of the performer."
—Samuel Johnson

First, you must know WHAT you are dealing with and if it is dementia. Now, we introduce some strategies relating to HOW to care for a person with dementia. It is impossible to cover every situation that may arise, but some general principles improve life for everyone involved. We also share examples to which you might relate or from which, you might extrapolate. Note that these are guidelines, not rules. Every individual is distinct and every situation individual. And, none of us is perfect. In fact, one of the most important themes in dementia care is flexibility. It all boils down to:

The seven common senses of dementia care

1. Respect
2. Teamwork
3. Routine
4. Preparation
5. Flexibility
6. Positive engagement
7. Safety

First Principle: Independence and Respect

Honoring the best interests of a person is the foundation of caregiving. For a family caregiver this means caregiving as an expression of love without oversmothering ("If it ain't broke, don't fix it."), but with recognition of when to step in and help, particularly when someone's health, safety, and well-being are at stake. Achieving

A.M. Lipton and C.D. Marshall, *The Common Sense Guide to Dementia*
for Clinicians and Caregivers, DOI 10.1007/978-1-4614-4163-2_6,
© Springer Science+Business Media, LLC 2013

this delicate balance is definitely easier said than done—BUT, it can be done! Like most things in life, practice and experience help, as does education in a variety of forms and talking to trusted others (which might include friends, family, fellow caregivers, and professionals. The latter could be your loved one's doctor or your own doctor or therapist). Respect not only a person's wishes but also their limits—and your own!

Determining a person's best interest should emphasize autonomy, whenever possible. This means letting each individual do and decide what they can for themselves and stepping in only as necessary. Avoiding present or future harm, not just physical but emotional and financial as well, is key in this determination. Try not to test a loved one at home (e.g., asking memory questions, such as "What is the date?"). Leave that for the doctor's office. Instead, determine a loved one's preferences from day-to-day life and your knowledge of the person, and use these as your guide. Can you work with as a team in managing finances if your husband likes to be involved, rather than having to take over completely? What does Mom enjoy doing? If she can't drive, arrange alternate transport to her bridge group. If she can no longer play cards, but still enjoys spending time with her friends, see if they be willing to have her join them for coffee afterwards.

Also, respect yourself as caregiver. It may be the best job you ever have. Caregiving is hard, but it can also be rewarding and empowering. So, respect your limitations, but also remember the valuable and often essential role you play in someone's life. If you can't think of a solution, talk to someone you trust and brainstorm together. The idea that two heads are better than one leads us to our second guiding principle:

Second Step: Teamwork

We've said it before, but can't say it too much: Care for the Caregiver. Help the Helper. Work as a Team. In addition to the individual needs of the patient with dementia, we must respect the tough job done by caregivers day in and day out. We have encountered many caregivers who feel they "must" go it alone. This attitude is not helpful and may be harmful in creating social isolation for the person with dementia and caregiver alike. Numerous studies show that social activity benefits mental and physical health. This includes people with dementia—and their caregivers, too.

For a patient with dementia who lives at home, a primary family caregiver who lives with (or close) to the patient might provide day-to-day care. Others involved may be family, friends and neighbors, and professional caregivers (via adult day programs or home care. A variety of options are discussed in detail in Chap. 15: Selecting Level of Care). As previously discussed, the patient should have at least one general physician and a dementia specialist (such as a geriatric psychiatrist or behavioral neurologist) may be extremely helpful. Play to the strengths of your team and delegate responsibility (especially jobs that you'd rather not do). Let the grown kids who are good on the computer manage online banking and prescription orders. And, avail yourself of advice and help from fellow caregivers, as well as the plethora of community and online resources from the Alzheimer's Association and other organizations.

If you are a caregiver and considering quitting work or another activity that you enjoy, this may mean that you need additional assistance from others. This could even be a sign of caregiver depression. Talk it over with others (see examples above), including your doctor and your loved one's doctor, too. See if you can find an alternate solution, including additional caregiving support. Maybe you'll still quit your job (that is, one besides your job as caregiver!), but maybe you will find that you don't need to stop working after all. Maybe your loved one enjoys the mental, social, and physical activities available in an adult day program while you are at the office. Of course, if you hate your job and have the financial wherewithal to quit, that's one thing, but, if you enjoy your work and only quitting because you think you "have to," that's another. At least consider trying additional caregiver support and/or a temporary separation (e.g., family leave) to see how things go before quitting your job completely.

And, if you are considering quitting a beloved activity that has been a cornerstone of your routine (anything from a social group to exercise to a hobby), this strongly indicates a need for additional caregiving support. Such a sacrifice doesn't help you—or your loved one. In fact, it only hurts by depriving you of an important outlet for diffusing stress and can create feelings of resentment regarding your caregiving responsibilities. It's not healthy. If you feel bad or guilty about taking a break, remember that your loved one may need a break from you, too! Since caregiving is more than a full-time job, it helps to have someone (or more than one) who you know and trust, is good with your loved one, and able to step in and help out when you can't due to life's little—and big—interruptions. Speaking of disruptions to routine brings us to the third Common Sense of Dementia care.

Third Thing to Do: Stick with It!

As we all know, life is often not routine, and things happen! That will be covered more in the next section. However, structure and routine represent critical components of dementia care.

Having a routine doesn't have to be boring, nor does it mean that you have to do the same thing everyday. It's often helpful to schedule two or three activities during the day, but these can be different activities, such as walking or other exercise, hobbies, and social activities. Perhaps a friend is available for lunch every Tuesday and you and your loved one go to the movies (or see one at home) on Fridays. Also, remember to think about space as well as time. Have a hook or basket near a door for keys. Have a set place for purses and wallets.

But, some things are better when done the same way at the same time each day. These include our basic functions and activities such as eating, sleeping dressing, and bathing. You don't have to eat the same thing each day, but it is helpful to have standard mealtimes. Similarly, with sleep, the quality of everyone's sleep (patient and caregiver/s) will be maintained or improved by set times. This includes a fixed bedtime as well as a routine time to wake up. A person's routine or preferences can easily be incorporated at home or in a long-term residential care situation. Sometimes you just have to ask. (What time does Dad prefer to wake up and how can we make that happen?) Having a set bedtime routine (turning down lights, putting on soft music, changing into pajamas, rubbing scented lotion into hands, having milk and cookies or another snack) may also help ease the transition to sleep. A scheduled post-lunch "siesta" may work better than allowing someone to doze off randomly during the day.

Scheduled voiding (i.e., taking a person to the bathroom at regular intervals) has been scientifically shown to minimize urinary incontinence ("pants-wetting") [1, 2] and often works better for patients with dementia than any bladder medication (as the problem is more about the "brain" aspect of urinary control than the bladder. Furthermore, as discussed in Chap. 8, many such medicines impair memory). Try taking your loved one to the bathroom based on their usual routine or else try once an hour and increase or decrease that time interval based on what works.

Speaking of incontinence, accidents can—and will—happen, along with lots of other bumps along the road, which brings us to our next point:

Fourth, Be Prepared

Don't just expect the unexpected, prepare for it. This includes holidays, hospitalizations, moves, guests, trips, and travel. Large gatherings and disruptions to routine may be disconcerting, to say the least, for a patient with dementia. Retain as much routine as possible. Make sure to have a quiet room that you can seek out if your loved one is overwhelmed by noise or crowds. Sometimes it's better to visit a loved one at home or other quiet, familiar place and one at a time, or in small numbers. If you've followed our previous advice about carrying a list of a patient's medications (see Chap. 4), you're that much more prepared for any hospitalization or other medical procedure—or trips. If you don't think that your loved one will travel again, make sure to have a care plan if you're sick or called away. This might include lining up a family caregiver, a professional in-home caregiver, or respite care at a residential facility. Have your loved one's doctor complete any required medical forms, exams, orders, and tests (e.g., for tuberculosis, "TB"), and do this now rather than rushing around at the last minute when you might also be preparing for a last-minute trip or be unable to do so due to other circumstances (e.g., should you fall ill and/or require hospitalization).

Many patients with mild or even moderate dementia can travel well in the company of a caregiver. However, prepare for possible disorientation and sleepless nights given the departure from the usual routine. (Sleeping—and waking up—in an unfamiliar place and being thrown out of our usual routine can be difficult—and even transiently disorienting—for those of us without memory loss, so you can imagine how hard it may be for someone with even mild dementia.)

Your loved one may require additional assistance. For safety's sake, it's often wise to travel with at least one person of the same gender as the person with dementia, in case family bathrooms are not available. Check with your loved one's doctor, but, even if a physician approves, you need to consider travel plans carefully. Your loved one shouldn't go if it will cause more harm than good for the patient, you, and/or others.

If your loved one hasn't traveled for some time, it may be best to start with a short trial vacation close to home. If flying, you may want to have a letter from a doctor explaining that your loved one needs to travel with you and may have difficulty answering security questions due to memory loss. (Airport security required one of our patients to proceed through a separate security line from his wife despite her explanation that he had Alzheimer's disease and they needed to stay together. The security agent reportedly said, "He looks fine to me.")

Have a "dummy" or duplicates for items such as wallets and purses that are frequently misplaced (and, of course, nothing of significant value, including identification, insurance, and credit cards, or large amounts of money, should be kept in them, if these are often lost). This also applies to glasses, make-up lipstick, and the like. If the toothpaste tube always goes missing, buy travel sizes. Be prepared and be creative, which brings us to our next point:

The Fifth Element: Flexibility

It isn't common sense to do the same thing over and over and expect a different result. Alter course when something doesn't work. Don't beat your head against the wall repeatedly. Don't beat your head against the wall repeatedly. Don't beat your head against the wall repeatedly.

Try another tactic: Rest, hugs, distraction (snack, car ride, other activity), leave a room and return in a few minutes. Count to 10—or 100! Use memory loss to advantage, not disadvantage. For example, depending on the degree of a person's dementia, they might be perfectly happy and occupied by activities that might seem tedious or boring to someone with normal memory. Gear such tasks to the person's likes and level of ability. These might include sorting playing cards, sweeping or vacuuming, or stuffing envelopes. It might also include folding the same basket of clothes over and over or reading the same magazine again and again. We're sure you can think of many more, and, especially, know of things that your loved one specifically enjoys doing.

If a loved one has asked you what the date is 3 times in 1 min, you should be looking for a pen and paper to write it down. Or a calendar on which to show them. Or thinking about buying a large wall calendar and/or dry erase whiteboard, so that you can easily display and direct them to this information each day.

You don't have to be a genius to be ingenious. And, if you feel frustrated or annoyed or like you have a problem that you can't solve, look to others for support (remember, we're a team).

The Sixth "Common Sense": Positive Engagement

"You never win an argument with a patient with Alzheimer's Disease." This frequently applies to people with other types of dementia as well, since memory, judgment, and abstract reasoning worsen as dementia progresses. Therefore, it is best to avoid direct confrontation. To put it bluntly, don't start an argument. Go along. Go with the flow. Try agreeing! Show, don't tell. Long explanations are usually not the answer. Words of reassurance and support may be.

If a person with dementia hallucinates at night, seeing nonexistent "strangers" are in the house, it usually does not work to deny the hallucination outright and just say that no one is there. The "strangers" may be scary and real to your loved one. Try different strategies such as a reminder that you're here and that the doors are locked and it's safe. Point out the phone by the bed.

Just as you can show rather than tell, it's often better to do, than tell—and often to do with your loved one. If an item like a wallet is misplaced, it may help to look for it together. For the example of nighttime hallucinations above, if verbal reassurance doesn't work, try turning on lights, asking where the "strangers" were, and checking with your loved one to make sure "they're gone." Perhaps make checking door locks together before you go to bed part of your nightly routine. If you have another technique that works, by all means stick with it (until or unless it doesn't routinely work).

Avoid what doesn't succeed and embrace what does. In case of a potential argument brewing, agree, tell a funny story (it helps to have a few ready or carry a joke book), or change the subject (using memory loss to advantage). Sometimes no words at all will help. But other approaches may. These include hugs and distraction via an activity, which might include a snack, calling a beloved friend or relative on the phone, listening to favorite music, watching a TV program, crafts, household tasks, and many, many more—probably even more than you can think of yourself. Ask your loved one what he or she would like to do. You can also get ideas from friends, families, fellow caregivers, the Internet, and books (this book lists a variety in previous chapters as well).

Let your loved one with dementia be your guide. Enter their world. Remember that patients with Alzheimer's disease often recall the past better than the present. Therefore, if they wish to speak of dead relatives as if they were still alive or past events as if they are ongoing, it's OK for them—and you!—to do so. (Of course, if it's upsetting change the subject or activity.) When it comes to music, play or sing favorite "golden oldies." Reminiscing over old family pictures or photo albums can be a wonderful activity and generate many others. You may even want to display some of these or make a memory book of favorite photos (or copies) with brief explanations of each. Some patients with dementia forget their age and may not recognize their own reflection, expecting to see a much younger person. Consider removing or covering mirrors to avoid this upset. Television newscasts can be extremely unsettling to patients with dementia, particularly if they believe a news story like a fire is happening to them then and there. The TV can be removed or unplugged or you might take advantage of the many recorded programs now widely available to watch old or new favorite musicals, TV series, and movies that delight rather than disturb.

Tailor activity for the interests and ability level of the person with dementia. Set your loved one up for success, not failure. Maybe your wife used to be a great cook, but now forgets ingredients. If dinner is a disaster, have a laugh over it, rather than a blow-up. Cook with her. Step in (or take over) as needed for any frustration or safety concerns, while allowing her to perform the steps that she can do safely and stress-free. If she used to make dishes from scratch and now becomes easily confused, see if she can follow a recipe. Help recreate favorite dishes or find similar ones from her recipe box, family members, cookbooks, or the Internet.

Above all, don't critique people with dementia. It's not their fault. They can't help it if they forget or lose something. And, remember the "short-term" memory goes first in Alzheimer's Disease and most dementias. So, instructions or directions are likely to be quickly forgotten, although emotional upset may persist. (If a problem occurs, it's much better to find another way to prevent this from happening again rather than assigning responsibility or blame.) Maybe your loved one put the ice tray in the pantry rather than the freezer, but reminding him or her will only make you both feel bad.

You may be right, they may be wrong, but agreeing to save the peace is often a better approach in the long run than proving your point. However, we are all imperfect and the daily frustrations of caring for a loved one with dementia can be many. If you do or say something you regret, try to defuse the situation as quickly as possible. Provide reassurance. Forgive yourself and try to do better next time (and do what you can to prevent a "next time"). If you find that you are more irritable on a regular basis, consider additional caregiving assistance and even whether you need to speak with your own doctor or therapist about the demands upon you. Give yourself and your loved one a break—maybe even a snack break. You may never win an argument with a person with dementia, but most of them love a treat. And, you may deserve one, too.

Although it's best to avoid confrontation and usually best to honor a person's wishes, a line must be drawn when it comes to protecting the safety of your loved one and others. Sometimes it is not possible to agree with someone with dementia who puts themselves and/or others in harm's way:

The First and Last Common Sense: Preserving Safety—and Sanity

Believe it or not, hearing that they have Alzheimer's disease (or another type of dementia) is not the most disturbing thing for most of our patients, hearing that they can't drive is.

Even though this is the last section of this chapter, safety, is, of course, always first. Preserving safety and sanity for all is critical for patients with dementia and caregivers alike. As mentioned at the beginning of this chapter, one of the most important components of caregiving is knowing when to stand back and when to step in. That is, knowing when to say when.

And, if you aren't sure whether your loved one with dementia can safely drive, live alone, walk unaccompanied, cook, possess a firearm, drink alcohol, etc., such doubt can be a pretty good indicator that they shouldn't be. Studies show that a patient with dementia is generally not a good judge of whether or not he or she is safe to drive), but that caregivers of patients with dementia are much better able to determine whether or not a patient is safe to drive [3]. When it comes to driving or any other activity that should be more closely supervised, curtailed, or stopped altogether, utilize the sensible strategies outlined in this chapter to help find a creative way to do so in a manner acceptable to the patient and others. Use the "start low and go slow" principle in providing care. First, monitor daily activities. Address any problems with appropriate and specific intervention. These may include supervising, limiting, or stopping activities. It might also mean doing things together. A pattern of problems (repeated or similar problems) with a given activity should raise red flags indicating a need to step in.

For example, if a person with dementia becomes lost with driving, consider the context in deciding what to do next. Was the person driving to a very familiar place, such as someplace they go daily or weekly? If so, at a minimum, this person shouldn't drive alone and maybe shouldn't be driving at all (again, consider all the circumstances, including driving skills, which should be regularly monitored by family and/or formally tested). If a driver with dementia becomes lost going to a less familiar place, driving alone may be problematic. Is this someone who uses (not just possesses!) a mobile phone and could call for help? However, keep in mind that mixed messages may be hard to keep straight. Sometimes, it is easier on everyone for a person with dementia to stop driving altogether rather than setting particular—and possibly confusing—restrictions about area, time of day, driving accompanied or alone. Someone who routinely becoming lost shouldn't drive. Someone who has problems with driving skills or obeying traffic laws shouldn't drive. Someone who has problems driving in their own driveway or neighborhood shouldn't drive. The question is, does this apply to someone you know?

It sometimes helps to take a step back and try to view things a bit more objectively (or check with someone else who can, such as another family member or a doctor). Take the "next-door neighbor" or "grandchild" test: What action do you think should be taken if you heard that someone else's spouse or parent having the problems that your loved one is having with an activity? In terms of driving, would you feel safe riding in the car with that person? Would you let a child you know ride in the car with that person? Would you want that person driving in the neighborhood in which that child plays? Remember driving does not occur on a closed course, but on an actively changing one.

We often hear something along these lines from family caregivers for patients who have dementia severe enough to make driving unsafe:

> Dad doesn't understand why he can't drive. We argue about it all the time. And he gets mad when I remind him that his doctors told him to stop driving. Would you please explain it to him again?

First, don't argue! You'll lose. Second, recognize that the problem here may not be limited to memory. Insight, judgment and problem-solving may also be impaired. Dad may not remember his physicians restricting his driving, but repeated reminders, explanations, and discussion are unlikely to be beneficial and may instead be met with anger and frustration. As noted in the study mentioned above, patients with dementia generally don't recognize their own problems with driving. Dad likely feels he drives well even with evidence to the contrary. Patients with dementia may try to explain away multiple motor vehicle collisions or episodes of becoming lost as if family, doctors, or others are overreacting. Many express feelings of being unjustly targeted.

If you don't think your loved one with dementia is safe to drive, you should take action to address this, including informing his or her physician. In Chaps. 4–5, we discussed how it may be helpful to give the doctor a note at the appointment with information and updates on patient problems. Such a note is usually a better way to convey driving difficulties, as most patients become upset if these are mentioned, let alone discussed.

So, if your loved one with dementia is no longer safe to do drive, you should avoid raising the subject. In case he or she brings it up, have such a short, stock answer at the ready and repeat if necessary—or write it down. You might ask the doctor to write a "prescription" indicating that the patient should not drive (don't post this, just pull it out as needed). Whatever you do, pick one explanation and avoid a long discussion. Then, change the subject or try to employ a distracting activity. We readily acknowledge that this subject may be one of the hardest (in the world) from which to successfully disengage.

When it comes to loss of driving privileges, many of our patients are more accepting of reasons other than memory problems or poor driving performance. Some medical justifications that may be more palatable include poor eyesight or pain or weakness in arms or legs. You might even assign the blame to a physician to take the onus off of you. "Dad, the doctor said you are not allowed to drive. I am sorry but there is nothing I can do." We have had family members employ a variety of successful strategies with loved ones with dementia who shouldn't be driving: explaining that insurance is now unaffordable or canceled, hiding keys, disabling the car, or sending it for "repair" to "the shop" (at which there is an endless "waiting for the part," if the car's absence is noted). Sometimes keys must be secured and/or engines disabled to prevent unsafe driving of shared vehicles. But, if Dad's car is not needed for others to drive him, we advise removing it from the property to minimize a very large visual trigger. A good rule of thumb is not to have more cars than drivers and not to routinely park within easy eyesight of the household of a person with dementia who can't drive (i.e., park inside a garage, rather than on the driveway). If you can't keep a vehicle "out of sight, out of mind," an unsafe driver must still be kept off the road.

For a loved one who remains adamant about driving, you might request a referral from the doctor for comprehensive neuropsychological evaluation and/or a formal driving assessment. Check with the physician to see if a local medical or rehabilitation center has a driving assessment program. This is used to assess driving abilities of brain injured patients (stroke, head injury, etc.), but can be applied to dementia. Keep in mind these assessments can be costly are not typically covered by medical insurance. A free option may be available at the Department of Motor Vehicles, but remember that such agencies are not generally equipped to assess complex cognitive function. Family and physicians can truthfully tell the patient that he or she can resume driving upon passing the assessment, but not until such time. If he or she then tries to engage in discussion about the unfairness of the restriction, you can respond with "The doctor said you could resume driving if you pass the assessment." It is certainly a more positive response, and takes a burden off of the caregiver, putting the ball in the patient's court. Frankly, many patients with dementia will just not follow through, perhaps due to an underlying fear of not passing. We recommend being cautious and not scheduling the assessment on the patient's behalf. If a patient doesn't have the cognitive wherewithal to make such an appointment, he or she should not be driving. If the patient passes the assessment, this provides a greater level of comfort to everyone in lifting the driving restriction. Family should continue to monitor the driving abilities of such a patient (including riding as a passenger at least every 2 weeks). If Dad does not pass the assessment, everyone can feel more confident with the restriction.

Some states require physicians to report any patients diagnosed with dementia or similar issues. However, an unsafe driver can be reported in any state to the appropriate agency by anyone, including a doctor. Of course, even a revoked driver's license may not stop some people from driving. Someone with dementia who has had his or her driver's license revoked and continues to drive may need to be moved to a secure (locked) memory care unit to prevent harm to self or others, if access to a car cannot be prevented another way,

Let us not forget that driving cessation often equates to loss of independence. Even when family and friends are available for transportation, Dad may not want to rely on them. It may be preferable to use a paid companion to do the driving.

It is always best to err on the side of safety. For the patient. And the caregiver. And the rest of us, too.

Summary

A common sense approach to caregiving implies a balanced approach with neither too much nor too little intervention. Respect, teamwork, routine, preparation, flexibility, taking cues from the person with dementia, and safety are sound principles that can guide caregivers to a workable solution for day-to-day problems. However, much caregivers strive to get things "just right," they should not expect to be perfect. There is no cure for dementia, but there are better ways to cope and care.

References

1. Skelly J, Flint AJ. Urinary incontinence associated with dementia. J Am Geriatr Soc. 1995;43:286–94.
2. Ouslander J, Schnelle J. Assessment, treatment and management of urinary incontinence in the nursing home. In: Rubenstein L, Wieland D, editors. Improving care in the nursing home: comprehensive review of clinical research. Newbury Park, CA: Sage Publications; 1993. p. 131–59.
3. Iverson D, Gronseth G, Reger M, et al. Practice parameter update: evaluation and management of driving risk in dementia. Neurology. 2010;74:1316–24.

Chapter 7
Caring for the Caregiver

We have a special message for caregivers: *Your loved one will only do as well as you are doing.*

A caregiver has to take care of himself or herself first in order to be ready, available, and healthy enough to assist another. If the caregiver's mental or physical health worsens, he or she may become unable to care for himself or herself, let alone the patient. So, if you're a caregiver, take care of yourself. This means seeing a primary care doctor and any other specialists necessary to ensure your overall health, educating yourself, and enlisting assistance when you need it. If you are overwhelmed, need some days off, or want a housekeeper, then by all means bring in help. This may include other relatives, friends, and/or professionals (medical and other). It also may mean going outside the home for planned respite care, in which your loved one might attend an adult day program or stay overnight (or longer) in a memory care unit or similar facility.

None of us want the caregiver to burn out. You don't need to act alone and it's actually much better not to try to fly solo. Remember that socialization benefits both patient and caregiver. Furthermore, working as part of a team also usually optimizes medical care. Speaking of which, even experienced and/or professional caregivers need to take heed of this advice. The more we mature in our caregiving skills, the greater our tolerance, but the lesser our awareness, of stress. If you are even contemplating whether you might need a hand, then it is worth at least looking into or inquiring about additional assistance. As long as financial considerations were taken into account, we have never heard of a caregiver who got help "too soon."

Common sense rule: A patient will only do as well as his or her caregiver does.

Family Members of Caregivers

This section is directed mainly to adult children of parents dealing with dementia, but other relatives and caregivers may certainly find it applicable as well.

A.M. Lipton and C.D. Marshall, *The Common Sense Guide to Dementia for Clinicians and Caregivers*, DOI 10.1007/978-1-4614-4163-2_7, © Springer Science+Business Media, LLC 2013

Physicians learn early in their training that an abnormal finding might be missed without thoroughly checking for it. This principle explains why we perform a history and physical in the methodical fashion outlined in Chap. 5. Such careful assessments are especially important for a slow-moving disease like dementia, which tends to sneak up on a patient (and family) little by little.

If you have one parent with dementia and one who is the primary caregiver, you need to monitor the situation, too. This is not only true for parental caregivers who have expressed problems but also for those who haven't. Caregivers may become so hopeless that they give up on any help or solution. They may feel too tired or overwhelmed to pick up the phone or converse in detail about what they are going through. They may also consider it a failing or find it embarrassing to mention such problems to others, especially their children. Therefore, you need to ask questions and also see how things are going with your own eyes.

Find out how your caregiver parent is doing, feeling, and coping. Learn about any particular issues that have emerged in caring for your family member with dementia in any of the "ABCs": Activities of Daily Living (ADLs), Behaviors, or Cognition. Ask about any depressed mood and any problems with sleep or appetite, which can be signs of depression. It's important to know about these issues in the caregiver as well as for the patient. Caregivers of patients with dementia suffer from depression at high rates, especially if the patient has depression and/or behavioral problems [1]. On a happier note, a variety of strategies, including caregiver education and support may be helpful [2] and even delay the placement of a patient into a nursing home [3, 4]. Physicians typically focus office assessments on cognition, but problems with ADLs and behaviors can impose significant daily difficulty for a family caregiver and, along with the caregiver's health, are major reasons for institutionalizing a loved one with dementia [5].

Common sense rule: Care for the primary caregiver.

If your caregiver parent hasn't asked you for help, ask your parent. If your parent declines your assistance, but you suspect it may be needed, express your interest in making life easier for them as subtly and unobtrusively as possible. Parents may be leery of getting help from their grown children, so it is often best to make it about you, rather than them. For example, if you would like to attend a doctor's visit, you might say that you have some questions that you would like to ask the physician and inquire as to whether you could go with them to the clinic to do so.

Make specific proposals of help, especially in ways in which you may be well-suited, such as making doctor appointments and/or driving your parents to these. For parents who are not as adept with computers, offer to convert ordering medications to online and manage these for them. Depending on the circumstances, it may also be helpful to do this with banking or other financial transactions.

Specific times and types of help work best. They are often more practical, easier to receive, and more likely to be accepted, while still offering flexibility. ("Mom, I have Thursdays off and I could take Dad out golfing that day. I could also take him out on the weekend.") This honors and respects an individual's ability to choose between a couple of good choices (or accept them all!). It usually works best to find nonthreatening approaches of assistance and avoiding blatant interference or injury to anyone's pride and dignity. If offers for help are declined despite an apparent obvious need, your options may include stepping in more assertively, enlisting other family members or friends, and/or consulting with your parents' doctors or other medical professionals.

Common sense rule: Make specific offers of help.

Adult children need to keep a close eye on a parent who is a caregiver to make sure Mom is taking care of herself or Dad has some help with the cooking or whatever the case may be. Our experience is that parents often minimize their caregiver burden to and decline offers of assistance from their grown children. Such spousal caregivers often express to us that they don't wish to "bother" their offspring and conceal their real level of distress. We therefore find it helpful to include the adult children (or at least one) at the clinic visit whenever possible.

You might spend a few days and nights staying with your parents quietly and unobtrusively observing how they do from day-to-day. If family members do not live close by or this is otherwise not feasible, consider hiring a geriatric care manager to perform an in-home assessment. It may work best to enjoy a social visit and avoid critiquing or intervening (unless a situation poses a basic health or safety risk), so that you can how things go when you're not there. Obviously, it is important to pitch in as needed, but it is also essential to observe the daily routine (or lack thereof) as it occurs when you're not present, so that you can see what works, what doesn't, and what might be improved.

You may be very surprised by what you find, so prepare yourself. For example, you might schedule a family meeting with your sibling or siblings, by phone or in person, to occur before and/or after the visit, so that you can talk things over. You might also need some time after your visit for reflection, research, or even just some relaxation.

Once you have assessed the situation in your parents' home, then you might develop a plan of action by meeting with your caregiver parent and/or other family. Of course, if you do perceive health or safety risks, these need to be addressed immediately as well as for the long-haul. If you conclude that your caregiver parent is struggling, intervene. The decline we see in a patient sometimes corresponds more to the caregiver's decline than due to the patient's underlying dementia. And, remember, sometimes the spouses of our elderly patients develop dementia, too. In fact, the spousal caregivers of patients with dementia have been shown to experience dementia at a rate six times higher than their age-matched peers [6], perhaps due to the difficult demands of caregiving for a loved one with a dementing illness.

Just because you aren't aware of a problem, doesn't mean it's not there. Look, listen, and dig deeper. Patients have regular examinations. Make sure to check the caregiver, too. Preventive care is always best. If a problem can't be completely avoided, perhaps it can be minimized.

Common sense rule: Live a day (or more) in a primary caregiver's shoes.

Caregiver and Family Dynamics

We conclude this chapter by pointing out problematic caregiver and family issues that we see regularly in caring for patients with dementia. We suspect that some of these difficulties reflect the underlying personality organization of the individual or a family member's internal struggles. Others represent family dynamics that eventually manifest in problematic caregiving behavior. No easy solutions exist for predicaments stemming from ingrained personality types and family dynamics. However, individual or group psychotherapy may sometimes help deal with these issues.

If any of these apply to you or your family, the first step is recognition. The second step is contemplation. Consider how you and your family might avoid or minimize conflict and counterproductive behaviors. Such measures might include counseling. It is unlikely that long-standing family or personality problems will be resolved. Stress and illness usually exacerbate these troubles rather than resolving them. Keep in mind as you read this section that each of us has flaws and almost every family has some level of dysfunction, but most caregivers that we encounter (especially unpaid family members) are good, well-intentioned, and altruistic individuals doing the best they can in a very sad, difficult, and challenging situation. So, caregiver, know thyself. But remember, the most likely answer to the question, "What kind of caregiver am I?" is "A good one."

Some Caregiver Types and Traits

We all have personality traits that can work to our advantage or disadvantage. For example, you probably want your doctor to be attentive to detail, and most doctors are, although you might also become frustrated by how long you must wait for one who takes his or her time. Such traits can influence what types of caregivers we are. Awareness of these can help you capitalize on your strengths—and minimize pitfalls.

The Inflexible Caregiver. This is someone who cannot adjust to the changes in a loved one (or life in general). The inflexible caregiver lives in a world of black and white. Instead of letting things slide, he or she feels compelled to correct each misstatement a patient with dementia utters. The inflexible caregiver doesn't appear to know what the term "roll with it" means. He or she would never even consider bending the truth for the greater good. Since flexibility is one of the main keys in living with a patient with dementia, this caregiver will be traveling a hard road.

Common sense rule: It is better to bend than to break.

The Micromanager. Often we see micromanaging as a way of dealing with the depression, anxiety, anger and/or guilt that caregivers experience. The Micromanager channels these feelings into creating documents and lists. He or she looks over the shoulders of all other caregivers, which might include the staff of a facility where a patient resides. The Micromanager calls the physician's office so often that the receptionist can identify his or her voice. We, as physicians, are often impressed by the thoroughness of the Micromanager. However, the Micromanager tends to take on too much alone and may lose the forest for the trees, rather than letting some things go in favor of more pressing issues. From a psychiatric standpoint, we want to make sure the micromanaging is not being used as a diversion to avoid experiencing the strong emotions that this disease can elicit.

A Micromanager needs to learn to delegate what, when, and where needed and have time and an outlet for diversion and relaxation.

> A woman in her 70s with moderate-to-severe Alzheimer's disease required 24/7 care, including assistance with dressing and bathing. They had no relatives nearby and her husband gave up his long-standing weekly tennis game despite repeated recommendations by her dementia specialist to obtain outside help (including professional help covered by long-term care insurance), so that he could resume this. He tried a couple of professional in-home caregivers but rejected each after one visit as he said that his wife didn't want anyone else but him to take care of her and that none of the aides lived up to his exacting standards. At each visit, the patient's husband provided a typed list of her medications and a detailed update on her condition, which was also typed out. She participated in a clinical research trial in which the study medication her husband administered to her was checked and counted at regular intervals, always with 100 % compliance. After several years, the patient's husband finally relented to having a part-time in-home professional caregiver (paid for by their insurance) and this appeared to be a good solution for both of them. The patient had always interacted well with all of our office staff and got along well with this companion from an outside agency, too. Her husband enjoyed going back to playing tennis regularly with his friends. He appeared more rested and relaxed and both seemed happier at clinic visits.

Common sense rule: Sometimes the patient needs a break from the caregiver!

The "I just want to make them happy" Caregiver. On the surface, there is nothing wrong with this attitude. However, it is concerning when taken to the extreme. It is relatively easy for a doctor to spot a patient that is hard (or impossible) to please. So, when we see a caregiver of such a patient jumping through hoops for naught, we will ask the caregiver about the fervor behind their efforts. Often the explanation given is to make the patient "happy." Typically, we ask the caregiver whether the patient has ever been happy. When the caregiver's response is to laugh at this notion, it becomes evident that even taking great pains to do so will remain futile. It is important to realize that ingrained personality traits are unlikely to change and may become even more pronounced in the case of dementia. In these types of cases, we do not want to see the caregivers set themselves up to fail.

Common sense rule: Don't bend over backwards for naught.

The Martyr. We recognize the significant sacrifices that all caregivers must make. However, the Martyr caregiver may dominate a doctor's visit or support group in talking about how overwhelmed he or she is, while categorically rejecting all recommendations and offers of assistance. Extreme sacrifice of one's interests for another (or others) may represent a long-standing role or personality trait. The Martyr caregiver may have built his or her life around the caregiving role, and this may comprise a significant part of his or her identity. Therefore, there may be considerable backlash against the intrusiveness of others, even if such action is required for the patient's (and caregiver's) well-being. We have seen success when other family members step in and put assistance in place (despite reluctance from the primary caregiver), while acknowledging the importance of the primary caregiver, preserving his or her sense of purpose, and involving him or her prominently in the patient's continuing care. The best strategy for dealing with dementia is a team approach. It serves no purpose to add to the suffering of this disease by rejecting help and trying to go it alone.

> A woman participated for the first time in a caregiver support group moderated by two dementia specialists. Her husband, who was 68 years old, had been diagnosed with "dementia" by the patient's general practitioner. She spoke about problems she was having caring for him, including some that posed risks to the patient and others. These included driving against medical advice and carrying around a loaded gun in his pocket (which had accidentally discharged into their refrigerator, but fortunately had not harmed the patient or any other person). This support group represented her first attempt to reach out for help beyond the patient's primary care doctor. During the rest of that day's session, all members of the group offered support to this caregiver and a variety of suggestions, all of which were rejected. Soon thereafter, other relatives of this patient stepped in to arrange his placement in a memory care unit where he stayed social and active.

Common sense rule: If it's broke, fix it.

Family and Caregiver Issues

Although we often see the following issues in the context of family dynamics, they certainly may apply to the individual caregiver as well.

Families Paralyzed with Indecision. We sometimes work with families who will discuss something to death, but never make a decision. We may be amazed to look back in the medical record and see that we've been discussing a particular topic for over a year without any progress. This may reflect underlying family dynamics. We have also witnessed some families so paralyzed that they actually try to defer all decisions to the person with advancing dementia. Calling a family meeting is a first step in addressing this problem. Depending on the patient's cognitive abilities, it may be necessary to have the family meet without the patient. If you have any questions about this, check with the patient's dementia specialist. Follow-up or regularly scheduled family meetings may be required, but if you have had a couple of such get-togethers without resolution of major issues, then consider scheduling a family appointment with a therapist and/or the patient's physician. Regularly scheduled doctor's visits (rather than just calling the clinic for help and/or making an appointment when a crisis arises) and following our tips to make the most of medical help, as outlined in the preceding chapters, can also be beneficial.

Common sense rule: Make decisions and follow through.

Family Members Trying to Settle Old Debts. Family relationships can be hard. Sometimes a spouse or a parent fell quite short of the ideal. What if Mom withheld love and approval or drank her way through your formative years? Maybe Dad was absent. Perhaps your spouse was unfaithful. Sometimes we work with families mired in the history of their relationship. One of the more common scenarios we see is an adult child seeking the love and approval of a parent who long withheld both. Even as a rational, high-functioning adult, it's difficult to resist the chance to finally meet that need. The idea is as follows: If I take good care of Mom during her decline, she will love and accept me. Mom will be thankful and acknowledge my contributions. Unfortunately most of these situations end in disappointment. If Mom did not have insight into the situation when her brain was at its best, she will certainly not at its worst. Be mindful that childhood losses and longings may rise up in full force when you become a caregiver for the one who didn't adequately care for you. Some see an opportunity to right a wrong. In these situations, we strongly suggest an individual therapist for the caregiver. Even if you have no interest in dredging up the past, you need support during this time.

We also commonly see conflict between two or more family caregivers which may include sibling conflict and/or other issues. Therapy is much more sensible (and usually cheaper) than legal alternatives. Maintaining rapport is often the best way to avoid another party from engaging in legal action. Another option is to hire a geriatric care manager to serve as the point person in Dad's care. The care manager not only ensures Dad's needs are met, but can moderate between various family members who may have varying opinions on what is going on and what should be done about it.

If you are a patient's primary caregiver, reach out to and maintain lines of communication with other relatives. This might be through regular family meetings, phone calls, and/or email. Notify and invite immediate family to doctor's appointments. Find ways of engaging family members that wish to be involved (sometimes people are flattered just to be asked and certainly if you ask their input into how they might help). If you have any specific needs that you know would be aligned with their time, interest, and abilities, you might ask if they could help with those (such as asking your sister, who works with computers, if she could help your with ordering your mom's medications online).

We suggest that if you find yourself in a situation involving persistent unresolved conflict that you see a therapist—even if the other party won't.

Common sense rule: Don't use illness to settle old debts.

Denial. Denial is a part of life. We all regularly use some form of denial when assessing our beauty or golf game. However, in this case we're not talking about not being on the same page, we're talking about not being in the same book. Some families, even in advanced dementia, question whether their spouse or parent has dementia at all. This type of denial hinders families from moving forward and may even paralyze them into inaction. This is one of the most challenging parts of our work as dementia specialists. It is very hard to penetrate this defense mechanism and sometimes counterproductive to try. Fortunately, if you are reading this book, you are probably past this point.

If you are dealing with relatives who are in denial about a loved one with dementia, it probably won't work to "talk them out of it." You may wish to include them at visits with specialists or spend time with the patient, observing difficulties in performing daily activities, etc. Sometimes prolonged periods of time and/or significant crises may finally trigger a fuller realization of a dementia. Even in the face of forceful facts, denial is a powerful and often intractable defense mechanism. Most of our patients come to initial dementia evaluation after 2–3 years of decline in cognition, behavior, and daily function. In some cases, relatives only made appointment for their loved ones after a crisis (or repeated crisis) situation, such as being brought home by police after becoming lost or even jailed for disorderly conduct.

We are often asked about denial in patients with dementia. ("I think Dad is in denial about his memory problems.") This usually does not represent denial per se. Rather, it is very common for patients with mild dementia to have poor insight or awareness of their memory or other deficits rather than true denial.

Common sense rule: The first step towards a solution is acknowledging the problem.

Summary

Caregivers should consider their own mental and physical health and work as part of a team to optimize care for a patient with dementia. Family members should regularly monitor and check on loved ones with dementia and their primary family caregivers for stress and other quality of life issues and offer help. Personality types, defense mechanisms, and family history and dynamics may determine caregiving issues. These should be addressed if it is necessary and feasible to do so. Professional assistance, such as psychotherapy, may be indicated in some cases.

Common Sense Rules

- A patient will only do as well as his or her caregiver does.
- Make specific offers of help.
- Live a day (or more) in a primary caregiver's shoes.
- It is better to bend than to break.
- Sometimes the patient needs a break from the caregiver!
- Don't bend over backwards for naught.

- If it's broke, fix it.
- Make decisions and follow through.
- Don't use illness to settle old debts.
- The first step towards a solution is acknowledging the problem.

References

1. Teri L. Behavior and caregiver burden: behavioral problems in patients with Alzheimer disease and its association with caregiver distress. Alzheimer Dis Assoc Disord. 1997;11 Suppl 4:S35–8.
2. Sörensen S, Pinquart M, Duberstein P. How effective are interventions with caregivers? An updated meta-analysis. Gerontologist. 2002;42(3):356–72.
3. Gaugler JE, Roth DL, Haley WE, Mittleman MS. Can counseling and support reduce burden and depressive symptoms in caregivers of people with Alzheimer's disease during the transition to institutionalization? Results from the New York University caregiver intervention study. J Am Geriatr Soc. 2008;56:421–8.
4. Mittleman MS, Haley WE, Clay OJ, Roth DL. Improving caregiver well-being delays nursing home placement of patients with Alzheimer's disease. Neurology. 2006;67:1592–9.
5. Buhr GT, Kuchibhatla M, Clipp EC. Caregivers' reasons for nursing home placement: clues for improving discussions with families prior to the transition. Gerontologist. 2006;46(1):52–61.
6. Norton MC, Smith KR, Østbye T, Tschanz JT, Corcoran C, Schwartz S, Piercy KW, Rabins PV, Steffens DC, Skoog I, Breitner JC, Welsh-Bohmer KA. Cache county investigators. greater risk of dementia when spouse has dementia? The Cache County Study. J Am Geriatr Soc. 2010;58(5):895–900.

Chapter 8
Dementia Medications

"Start low and go slow."

—Maxim of Geriatric Physicians

"But keep going!"

—Cindy D. Marshall, M.D.

In this chapter, we discuss proper medication administration and supervision for the patient with dementia. We review various medications, including cognitive enhancers, those which may help symptoms of dementia, those which may worsen such symptoms, and those which are purported to help—but generally don't. We also include some tips for helping to decide when a medication is beneficial—and when it is not helping and may even be worsening dementia symptoms.

A regular review of medications is a cornerstone in the ongoing management of dementia. Vitamins, supplements, herbal remedies, and other alternative therapies, as well as over-the-counter and prescription drugs, have risks and the potential for drug interactions, as well as benefits, as will be discussed in this chapter. We therefore recommend creating a very inclusive medication list (see also Chap. 4).

Common sense rule: All medications have side effects.

This chapter doesn't provide a detailed pharmacologic overview of dementia medications (and such reviews are available elsewhere [1, 2]). Nor, do we discuss medications in development or under study which may have wider future applicability, which again can be found via other resources, including online. Rather, we hope to provide practical clinical pearls regarding currently available medications for dementia, focusing on common issues that we have encountered as clinicians.

If you are a family caregiver, we are happy to broaden your knowledge about drugs for dementia, but don't be tempted to change a loved one's medications on your own. Drugs that affect the brain should be started or changed with close medical supervision, especially in the elderly, who may be particularly sensitive to potential risks. Physicians need to be informed about adverse effects a patient may be experiencing and can provide crucial input.

A.M. Lipton and C.D. Marshall, *The Common Sense Guide to Dementia for Clinicians and Caregivers*, DOI 10.1007/978-1-4614-4163-2_8, © Springer Science+Business Media, LLC 2013

Common sense rule: Make medication changes only with a doctor's supervision.

General Medication Guidelines for Caregivers of Patients with Dementia

Medication Administration

First use a pillbox. This should be filled and checked by a family member at least weekly ("Trust, but verify"). Keeping the pillbox in plain sight on the breakfast table or by a coffeepot, toothbrush, or other routinely used item may serve as a helpful reminder. If medications are taken more than once a day, we recommend using two or more weekly pillboxes (e.g., a yellow one in the AM and a blue one for PM medications) or a pillbox with multiple slots. Pillboxes also help signal when prescriptions need to be refilled. If mistakes are made, additional support and supervision (with each dose, if needed) should be provided.

We can all forget a pill, but medications should be supervised for anyone taking medication specifically for memory problems. In particular, when "short-term" or recent memory is affected, one may forget to take a pill (or forget that a pill has already been taken and take it again and this can happen repeatedly, even in the same day). And any medications, not just those for memory, may be over- or under-dosed or taken erratically. Furthermore, most medications prescribed for memory generally have few side effects when taken regularly, but, if taken sporadically, may fail to help memory and have significant side effects (especially gastrointestinal side effects, such as diarrhea).

We strongly recommend that family caregivers adopt a team approach and "take your medications together" to help remind each other, jointly filling and using their respective pillboxes. This is usually a much kinder, gentler, and palatable method than simply "supervising" your loved one. Even if you don't take medications, consider starting a daily multivitamin or other vitamins (with your doctor's permission) as a show of support.

A 72-year-old woman was referred by her primary care physician to a dementia specialist for "possible" Alzheimer's Disease (AD) and inability to tolerate a drug prescribed for this due to diarrhea. She came to the clinic with her husband. They both reported that the patient took all of her own medications from the bottles. When making a list of medications for her appointment with the specialist, her husband had discovered that his wife had two bottles of the same prescription from different doctors and had probably been taking both. The dementia specialist counseled them regarding the patient's medication. Both were agreeable to filling and using pillboxes together. The patient was then able to tolerate the drug for dementia without difficulty.

Common sense rule: Use a pillbox and increase supervision as needed.

This case example also underscores our prior recommendation that a caregiver should have an accurate medication list and bring this to any medical visit as discussed in the preceding chapters. Such an inventory allows the physician to see if any drugs are redundant, unnecessary, or deleterious, as well as to check what additions might benefit the patient and any drug–drug interactions. It also helps a dementia specialist if you are aware of the names, dosages, and side effects of any medications for dementia that the patient has tried previously.

Medication Information and Side Effects

Medication information can be obtained from a variety of resources, including the prescribing physician, other doctors, nurses, pharmacists, printed material (including pharmacy information and manufacturer's inserts), and online. In our experience, such details can overwhelm many patients and families, so focus on main points from trusted sources (i.e., You can find anything on the Internet, don't read or believe all of it!).

We recommend that family caregivers discuss any medication with the prescribing physician, read over any printed (or similar online) information from the pharmacy, and also consult with the pharmacist, if needed. Usually reviewing such printed material once is sufficient. Familiarize yourself with the highlights and retain it for future reference. If you find yourself reading the details over and over, ask yourself if this is really helpful. In our experience, it usually isn't. It may actually be harmful in creating undue anxiety. We recommend focusing one's time, energy, and effort on caregiving for the patient, not the paper (or the computer screen). (Because learning new information is generally difficult for patients with dementia, we recommend even more strongly that they channel their energies elsewhere.)

Of course we want family caregivers to educate themselves, but we don't want them to worry excessively about this information (e.g., trying to memorize the entire list of side effects, etc.). Knowing the finer points of a medication is the job of the prescribing physician, who should certainly be consulted in case of a new or worsening problem occurring after the initiation of a medication. If there's something you don't understand, then by all means check with the pharmacist and/or prescribing physician. For substances not requiring a prescription, check with a patient's specialist, if possible, and/or family doctor regarding potential drug interactions, benefits, and risks.

Common sense rule: Be familiar with medications but most familiar with your medical team.

Due to the potential for drug–drug interactions, it is usually prudent not to start more than one medication at a time. Otherwise, if a patient has a subsequent ill effect, it may be unclear if which drug, drugs, or interaction thereof might be culpable and all may need to be withdrawn. Or, if a patient does better, both medications might be continued, when one could do the trick, creating additional cost and posing the potential for increased adverse effects and drug–drug interactions.

The same logic holds for stopping medications. If you stop more than one medication and a patient declines, how will you know which one should be restarted? Furthermore, just as neurologists and geriatric psychiatrists "start low and go slow" when initiating medications, when it becomes necessary to withdraw a drug (or drugs), we often prefer to similarly withdraw them slowly. Many neuropsychiatric medications (drugs that act on the brain) may have serious side effects if stopped suddenly.

Common sense rule: Don't start (or stop) more than one medication at a time.

It's a good rule of thumb not to start medications during major transitions. Change is hard, but even more so for patients with dementia. Even something usually considered to be a positive change, such as holidays, vacation, or hosting visitors, may be difficult for a patient with dementia. It may be logistically difficult (e.g., to reach a doctor or regular caregiver or obtain a new prescription) during travels or holidays, if a patient begins having symptoms associated with starting a new drug. We generally recommend that medications should not be changed within a couple weeks of a move or other transition for patients with dementia. Of course, there are exceptions to every rule and care should be individualized, especially if there is an imminent need to treat a medical issue (which might include behavioral problems in the case of dementia). Still, even if a patient is hospitalized, it usually makes sense to continue his or her usual medications unless a compelling reason exists not to do so. If medications for dementia are stopped for more than a few days, they are usually reintroduced at the starting dose and must be gradually titrated up (increased) to the maximally effective level.

> An 78 year-old woman diagnosed with AD one year previously by her family physician was brought by her son to a dementia specialist due to significant worsening since she moved into a memory care unit one month prior. Her dementia medications were stopped at the time of this move. In the past two weeks, the patient had been having daily episodes of agitation (despite no previous history of this) and was having more difficulty dressing herself. Over the next few months, the dementia specialist gradually added back the patient's medications, and the patient's agitation resolved. Her dressing ability also improved but not to the level she was functioning at prior to her move.

Common sense rule: Don't change medications during major transitions or disruptions to routine.

Off-Label Usage

If a drug lacks FDA approval for a particular medical condition, it may be because it is not effective in that specific situation. However, sometimes lack of such approval may simply mean that not enough research has been done and/or submitted to the FDA to meet its rigorous requirements. Because such studies and submissions are laborious and expensive, they may not be done even if some evidence indicates that a drug may be worth trying for a given disease state. Therefore, physicians sometimes prescribe medications which have been approved by the FDA as safe and effective for at least one medical reason in an "off-label" fashion if they perceive a possible indication (medical rationale) that may not be recognized by the FDA. Since there are no FDA-approved medications for many types of dementia and related symptoms, use of any drug to treat these conditions is by-definition "off-label." For example, a doctor may prescribe a drug with FDA approval for AD for another type of dementia. Furthermore, due to the paucity of drugs that are FDA-approved, we and other physicians sometimes prescribe medications that are FDA-approved as safe and effective for a condition other than dementia in an "off-label" fashion to treat dementia and its symptoms.

Cognitive Enhancers

The main medications presently available for the primary treatment of dementia are often called cognitive enhancers. (This may be somewhat of a misnomer, as we will discuss further.) Unfortunately, only two classes of medications are FDA-approved to treat dementia and all but one are indicated for Alzheimer's disease alone. Rivastigmine is the exception as it also has FDA approval to treat Parkinson's disease dementia (PDD). Therefore, at the time of writing this book, no medications are FDA-approved for any other types of dementia (like Vascular dementia or Frontotemporal dementia (FTD)). Furthermore, one class of these medications consists of just one FDA-approved medication (memantine, trade name: Namenda), which is only FDA-approved for the treatment of moderate-to-severe AD. The manufacturer's insert for each of these products contains full prescribing information (and are available online), but we share in this section some important highlights as well as some helpful tips based on our on real-world experience prescribing these medications.

Unfortunately, there is no cure for dementias such as AD. Furthermore, although the medications to treat dementia are called "cognitive enhancers," we don't typically expect them to result in dramatic improvements. Current medications generally treat symptoms of dementia and may also delay or slow decline in terms of cognition, behavior, function, or the patient's overall condition [1, 2]. Cognitive enhancers may also postpone nursing home placement [3] or save money on other aspects of medical care [4, 5]. You can think of the "*ABCDs*" of dementia treatment goals: *A*ctivities of Daily Living, *B*ehavior, *C*ognition, and *D*elaying institutionalization and possibly decline.

Because dementia is such a slow-moving disease, it may be difficult to appreciate this "slowing of decline" for an individual patient. Even if a patient with dementia wasn't on medication, we wouldn't expect to see much change over a time period shorter than months. Therefore, it is important to give cognitive enhancers a fair trial over at least a few months (so long as the patient isn't having any ill effects from them or there exists any other superseding reason to stop). It is also essential to titrate (gradually increase) to an effective or maximally effective dosage which generally takes at least a few weeks or even months. Despite these considerations, we often encounter cases in which doctors and/or family caregivers have stopped the patient's medication for dementia because the patient "didn't improve" even after trying just a starting dose for a short interval. An unfortunately all-too-common example illustrates this point:

> An 84 year old man was brought by his daughters to an initial consultation with a dementia specialist, who confirmed the patient's prior diagnosis of AD by his internist. That doctor had prescribed various drugs for AD, but the patient's daughters said that they stopped each of these after a few weeks as "nothing helped." The patient was living with one of his daughters as he was no longer able to live independently, but he still enjoyed walking daily. The dementia specialist counseled them regarding AD, available treatment options and expected results. She recommended restarting one of the medications for AD that had been previously tried and suggested that the daughters compare the patient's decline over the prior months (when he was not taking such drugs) to his daily function, behavior, and cognition over the next few months. All agreed that maintaining his exercise routine (with supervision) was an important goal of therapy. Over the next few months, his daughters noted that his overall decline had slowed, especially with regard to his activities and behavior. During this time frame, the dose of the cognitive enhancer was gradually titrated to a maximal dosage frame and another class of dementia medication was subsequently added and similarly increased. The patient was able to continue living at home with his daughter and walking with one of his daughters or another companion for the next couple of years.

Common sense rule: Don't stop a dementia medication due to "no change."

In the treatment of dementia and many chronic illnesses, we must manage our expectations and not expect a cure or even improvement. Our goal is to maintain our patients' living skills and slow symptom progression. We understand the frustration of patients, families, and other professionals that these medications do not offer more than they do. We feel the same way. However, we would choose symptomatic relief or the possibility of slowing of decline over a certain decline any day. These medications may provide financial savings to a patient, family, and society, as well as reduced caregiver burden. Why? Because with these medications, a patient may function at a higher level, have fewer behavioral problems, and live at home longer than without them. And, you cannot put a price tag on the internal and familial rewards that come along with that.

Cholinesterase Inhibitors

Several medications specifically approved by the FDA to treat dementia are classified as Cholinesterase (pronounced: cole-in-Esther-ace) Inhibitors: donepezil (trade name: Aricept), galantamine (trade name: Razadyne), rivastigmine (trade name: Exelon), and tacrine (trade name: Cognex). Tacrine is now rarely used due to its side effects and its requirement for frequent (four times a day) dosing.

A brain chemical (neurotransmitter) called acetylcholine is important in memory function. Acetylcholine decreases in AD [6] and as AD progresses [7]. Cholinesterase

Inhibitors (CIs) are designed to help maintain levels of acetylcholine in the brain, but do not address the other complex issues of AD or other dementia types, limiting the impact of CIs. They do not cure AD or other dementias. Rivastigmine is FDA-approved to treat PDD [8], but evidence exists for efficacy of donepezil in PDD[9]. Studies of galantamine in PDD are mixed [10, 11]. We generally prefer rivastigmine to the other CIs for patients with PDD due to the scientific evidence underlying its FDA approval. However, we have prescribed the other CIs (or kept patients on another CI as prescribed by another doctor) with results similar to that of rivastigmine. It should be noted that CIs may worsen motor features of Parkinsonism, such as tremor at rest, rigidity, bradykinesia (slowed movements), and postural instability (tendency to fall backwards).

Since reduction of acetylcholine is not a main feature of many non-AD types of dementia, CIs may not help people with a dementia other than AD. That said, CIs may help some individuals with other types of dementia. Therefore, due to the limited number of pharmacologic options, we often prescribe them "off-label" for patients with dementias other than pure AD or PDD We also sometimes do "off-label" prescribing of the medications approved for a given stage of AD in other stages of AD. That is to say, if a medication is FDA-approved only for mild-to-moderate AD, we may prescribe it "off-label" in moderate-to-severe AD, or vice versa.

In our clinical experience, agitation may sometimes occur (or preexisting agitation may worsen) after starting a CI in a patient with a non-Alzheimer dementia, such as FTD, Mixed (AD + Vascular) Dementia, and Vascular Dementia. However, we have prescribed CIs "off-label" for many such patients with good results, and most patients and families want to try this option, especially given the limited choices available.

Several studies have shown benefit for CIs in patients with Mixed Dementia or Vascular Dementia. The use of CIs in FTD is controversial (at least partially due to the lack of cholinergic deficit in this disease), but we have used them successfully, especially in language variants or motor presentations, such as Corticobasal degeneration (CBD) or Progressive Supranuclear Palsy (PSP).

We first treat any existing agitation (e.g., with an antidepressant type medication such as a Selective Serotonin Reuptake Inhibitor (SSRI)). If agitation occurs after starting a CI, we evaluate it on a case-by-case basis. We may add an SSRI or similar medication. We may also stop the CI, either temporarily or permanently, with strong consideration of the individual patient and family caregiver input.

We try to titrate (slowly increase) the dose of these medications to the maximum that a patient will tolerate (i.e., a dose a patient can take without experiencing significant adverse effects), especially as some evidence shows that increasing the dose more quickly may result in more side effects. Common side effects of CIs include nausea and diarrhea, but we find most patients tolerate these medications well if they are given with food and started slowly per the manufacturer's instructions (or even slower in some cases). Since many elderly patients suffer from constipation, we frequently find that CIs actually relieve this condition rather than causing frank diarrhea. A typical patient might have mild nausea and diarrhea for less than a week. We typically ask caregivers to monitor for side effects and call us if the patient has anything more than mild nausea and/or diarrhea and/or if these symptoms persist beyond a few days. We rarely receive such phone calls and, if so, usually do so in the face of mitigating factors, such as new infection and/or antibiotic (many of which can also cause nausea and diarrhea). In such cases, we usually recommend stopping the new CI until any infection resolves and the course of any antibiotic has been completed, at which time the CI can be reintroduced. If a patient has serious GI side effects including anorexia (reduced appetite/weight loss) or vomiting, we may switch to a different form (patch, liquid, or orally dissolving tablet) of the medication or stop it (temporarily or permanently). In our experience, patients particularly sensitive (or based on their medical histories predicted to be sensitive) to GI risks may do better if the CI is started after memantine (Namenda).

Fatigue is a possible side effect of CIs, but insomnia and nightmares or vivid dreams are as well (and usually more troubling for the caregiver and patient than fatigue). We find that these latter symptoms can usually be easily minimized by prescribing one of the once-a-day formulations ("off-label" in the case of donepezil) to be given in the morning after breakfast. In fact, we often avoid having to prescribe sleep aids to new patients with insomnia by simply switching their previously prescribed once-daily CI to be taken after breakfast or switching from a twice-daily preparation to a once-a-day preparation administered in the morning (again with food).

If a patient has heart or lung disease, CIs should be used with care. Bradycardia (slow heart rate), heart block, and syncope (fainting) are possible risks with any of the CIs, even in patients with no preexisting cardiac disease. Due to their mechanism of action, CIs may also exacerbate some types of pulmonary (lung) disease [such as asthma or Chronic Obstructive Pulmonary Disease (COPD)/emphysema].

Caution should also be exercised in prescribing CIs in other medical conditions which they may worsen, including bladder outflow obstruction and glaucoma.

We haven't seen any advantage in using more than one CI in an individual patient and prescription plan coverage of such a regimen may be difficult. Sometimes, families ask about any benefits of switching from one cholinesterase inhibitor to another. A lack of scientific evidence supports lasting effects of switching among these medications or preparations. And, our clinical experience is that there is not much point to switching among these medications or preparations unless the patient is unable to take a particular form due to a medical reason (having problems swallowing), noncompliance (not taking pills and medication must be crushed), or side effects (e.g., syncope). Hence, our practice is to select and continue the medication best suited to the individual patient and caregiving situation (e.g., if someone comes in to give the patient medications once daily, it doesn't make sense to start a twice-daily preparation).

Donepezil

Donepezil (trade name: Aricept) is FDA-approved for all stages of AD. It is available generically in 5 and 10 mg tablet form. Brand name (nongeneric) Aricept also comes in a 23 mg tablet. The manufacturer recommends that a patient take 5 mg daily for 4 weeks and to then increase to 10 mg daily and we adhere to this.

Our experience has been that it is difficult for patients to tolerate the doses higher than 10 mg due to gastrointestinal side effects, such as nausea, diarrhea, and vomiting. The manufacturer recommends that patients are on a 10 mg dose for at least 3 months before starting the 23 mg dose. If we plan to increase to 23 mg, we follow that rule, but then usually prescribe an even slower titration. We increase the dosage from 10 to 15 mg (usually one-and-a-half 10 mg tabs) daily for 1 month and then 20 mg (two 10 mg tabs) for a month prior to starting. Therefore, we do an "off-label" titration, even slower than recommended by the manufacturer to try to maximize the patient's chances of tolerating the medication (and to try to minimize any adverse effects).

With the exception of tacrine, which is no longer widely used, donepezil has been around longer than any of the other medications used to treat dementia. Ease of administration, including once-daily dosing, reduces patient and caregiver burden. Donepezil therefore has widespread clinical experience and acceptance and is the most commonly prescribed medication for dementia. The starting dose of donepezil is a clinically effective dose, so the patient is initiated straightaway on an efficacious dose.

These tablets may be crushed and put into food. They also may be split in half, if needed. Donepezil also comes in an orally dissolving tablet which may have to specially ordered, but can be helpful for patients who have difficulty swallowing pills.

The package labeling indicates that donepezil should be taken in the evening and may be taken with or without food. It is our general practice to prescribe it to be taken with food (to minimize potential gastrointestinal effects, such as nausea and diarrhea) and in the morning (to help avoid insomnia or vivid dreams/nightmares). Therefore, we usually prescribe donepezil "off-label" in that we usually prescribe it to be taken *after breakfast*. (If a given patient doesn't eat a good breakfast, then we usually recommend they take it after lunch.) Fatigue is a listed side effect, but, in our clinical experience, insomnia is more common.

Common sense rule: Adjust the timing of a medication to enhance normal sleep–wake cycle.

Galantamine (Reminyl/Razadyne)

If you or your loved one prefers natural remedies (or you are a doctor with a similar patient or family preference), note that galantamine is derived from the snowdrop, a flower similar to a daffodil.

Galantamine comes in a once-a-day capsule (8, 16, and 24 mg), twice-daily tablets (4, 8, and 16 mg), and liquid, and is available generically. We prefer to use once-daily dosing for ease of administration and enhanced compliance (it's much easier for a caregiver to give and a patient to take a medication once-a-day than twice a day). We have found galantamine in its liquid form to be a feasible option for patients who have difficulty with GI side effects, such as of nausea, diarrhea, poor appetite, and/or weight loss are unable to tolerate the patch form of a cholinesterase inhibitor (e.g., due to skin sensitivity).

Galantamine is FDA-approved for mild-to-moderate AD. We often maintain patients on this medication in an "off-label" manner as their AD progresses to mod-erate-to-severe, since at least one other CI (donepezil) has been shown to be beneficial in such cases, and we haven't seen benefit in switching among medica-tions in this class if a patient has done well on one (nor is their persuasive scientific evidence to support such a switch).

Common sense rule: Don't switch medications in the same class without good reason.

Rivastigmine (Exelon)

Rivastigmine (Exelon) can be taken as twice daily capsules by mouth or a patch applied to the skin. The capsules are available generically. Rivastigmine is the only FDA-approved medication to treat PDD. It is also FDA-approved to treat mild-to-moderate stage AD. Because the capsules come in many dosage strengths, rivastig-mine has the advantage of custom dosing but the disadvantage of having a complicated titration as the dose is increased. Also, the capsules require twice daily dosing (and should not be combined into a once-daily dosing as this could cause serious GI side effects). Even with twice daily dosing with food, patients may experience adverse GI effects, such as nausea, diarrhea, weight loss, and/or vomit-ing, especially at higher dosages. However, the capsules come in many different strengths making it easy to back down to a slightly lower dose to see if this will alleviate such effects.

The patch form of rivastigmine is quite useful for patients sensitive to any adverse effects from oral CIs. GI side effects, such as noted above, are possible with the patch, but much less likely since GI absorption is significantly bypassed. However, it takes more effort to apply the patch than just administering a pill. The patch may cause skin sensitivity, but in our experience, this is usually mild and the patch can often be continued with medical supervision of such sensitivity. It is important to follow the manufacturer's instructions on patch placement (it should be put on hair-less areas on the chest, upper arms, and back) and rotation (place a new patch in a different site daily, not to be applied to the same site within 14 days). Because of this regimen, a responsible person other than the patient should apply the patch.

To be sure and avoid a few common errors in patch placement that we have observed on a regular basis, we want to stress a few ways it should not be used. The rivastigmine patch should NOT be placed on the abdomen or buttocks, the same place each day, or kept on for more than a day. This could increase the chance for a skin reaction to the patch or other adverse effects.

We have found that rivastigmine capsules taken twice daily can be very helpful for patients with constipation, especially patients with Parkinson's disease for whom constipation may be a prominent or even the first symptom [12].

Common sense rule: Use side effects to a patient's advantage.

Table 8.1 Summary of Dementia Medication

Cholinesterase Inhibitors	FDA-approved pill forms	FDA-approved alternate forms
Donepezil (Aricept)	Once-daily tablet	Once-daily orally-disintegrating tablet
Galantamine (Razadyne)	Twice-daily tablets	Twice-daily oral solution
	Once-daily extended-release tablet	
Rivastigmine (Exelon)	Twice-daily capsule	Daily Patch, twice-daily oral solution
NMDA Antagonist		
Memantine (Namenda)	Twice-daily tablet*	Twice-daily oral solution

* A once-daily extended-release tablet is FDA-approved but not commercially available as of the time of the writing of this book.

For patients who are particularly sensitive to the GI side effects of a CI even when taken with or after a good meal, we generally either switch to the rivastigmine patch or memantine. Once memantine is titrated to its maximal dose, we may try an oral form of the CI again. This is because memantine may improve tolerance of a CI with fewer GI side effects (such as nausea and diarrhea).

Some patients have a significant GI history (e.g., extensive history of GI surgeries, Irritable bowel syndrome, etc.) or GI symptoms (e.g., nausea, diarrhea, poor appetite, and/or weight loss) even prior to starting a CI. In such patients, we generally prefer one of two options: either to first prescribe the rivastigmine patch or memantine. Again, once memantine is titrated to its maximal dose, we may try an oral form of the CI since memantine may improve tolerance as noted above (Table 8.1).

NMDA Antagonist

Memantine (trade name: Namenda) is the only medication in this class currently available and is FDA-approved for moderate-to-severe AD. Five and 10 mg tablets are available. It is usually titrated up to a goal dose of 10 mg twice daily over 4 weeks. We sometimes prescribe it "off-label" to be given once daily (two 10 mg tabs) for ease of use. It is dosed once daily in Europe and there is no pharmacologic reason to dose it twice daily (except if a patient experiences adverse effects). A once daily formulation (trade name: Namenda XR) has been approved by the FDA, but is not yet commercially available as of the writing of this book.

Listed side effects include constipation, dizziness, headache, and confusion. Although memantine can cause constipation, because it is often started after a CI (which tends to cause diarrhea), the GI effects often appear to "cancel each other out." Our practice is that if a patient has constipation, start with a CI first. Whereas for a patient who has a tendency toward diarrhea, we may prescribe memantine first.

Memantine, may cause dizziness or worsen preexisting symptoms of dizziness. In our clinical experience, headache and confusion rarely occur (and both usually instead improve) on memantine, whereas fatigue is somewhat common, but can be easily resolved by changing the dosage all to the evening.

Memantine is technically not supposed to be crushed as the tablets are film-coated but we are aware of cases in which this has been done without any apparent ill effects. It should be used with caution in patients with liver or kidney disease.

Off-Label Usage of Memantine for Non-Alzheimer Dementias

Although the FDA hasn't approved any medications for Vascular Dementia, a number of studies have shown that memantine is efficacious in this disease [13–16]. We have routinely prescribed memantine "off-label" to good effect for patients with Vascular or Mixed (Alzheimer's + Vascular) Dementia. We also often prescribe memantine in the case of PDD for which there is some evidence [17]. A larger study did not see the same effects in PDD, but did demonstrate the efficacy of memantine for DLB for which we also prescribe it [18], as well as for other Parkinson's-plus syndromes, such as CBD and PSP. CBD and PSP overlap with FTD as well as Parkinson's disease. Memantine has been studied in FTD [19], and we also use it in this condition.

Combination Therapy

The use of a CI and memantine together is called combination therapy and a number of studies have shown that these medications work well together, including with fewer GI side effect when combined [20–22]. It is our general practice to prescribe both of these medications for our patient with dementia, although we usually don't start them together.

We are aware of cases in which both memantine and a CI have been prescribed together by other physicians with no reported adverse effects. However, as aforementioned, it is not our general practice to start two medications separately due to the potential of drug–drug interactions and confusion regarding which drug, if any, might contribute to any adverse effects following simultaneous initiation.

In any dementia, either or both of these drugs are expected to provide symptomatic relief and may slow decline or stabilize the condition temporarily, but should not be expected to result in dramatic improvements. Unfortunately, but realistically, dementias like AD will continue to gradually worsen even with the best treatments currently available.

Common sense rule: Do not expect dramatic improvements.

Additional Medications for Dementia

Any and all vascular risk factors should be looked into and treated to the extent possible as these may worsen many different types of dementia. This includes Obstructive Sleep Apnea (OSA), which is an independent risk factor for stroke and can cause memory loss and fatigue. OSA is diagnosed via a sleep study and treated with a machine to keep airways open. Many patients with dementia may have difficulty undergoing a sleep study and/or using such a device, however, some patients with relatively mild attention and memory deficits primarily due to OSA may find significant relief of their cognitive problems. Medications for vascular risk factors might include antihypertensive medications for high blood pressure, statins for abnormalities of cholesterol and triglycerides (statins), cardiac medications for heart arrhythmias (including Coumadin/warfarin for atrial fibrillation), and oral antidiabetic medications and/or insulin for diabetes. Of course, prevention is the best medicine. Smoking is particularly dangerous for a patient with dementia due to the possibility of forgetting a lit cigarette and causing a fire and/or lacking the judgment to know what to do in case of a fire. Depression is a vascular risk factor, too, and can be addressed with medication and other means. This will be covered in chapters to come on mood and behavioral symptoms in dementia and treatment for these. Heart-healthy diet, exercise, and other activities (e.g., socializing) are all brain-healthy, too.

Common sense rule: What's good for the heart is good for the brain.

When to Stop Medication for Dementia

This is a common question in the severe or late stage of dementias which we also discuss in Chap. 16. It is important to regularly review medications for patients with dementia as their needs change and their response to the medication (both risks and benefits) may also evolve. Remember the ABCDs of dementia medication, delaying decline in Activities of Daily Living, Behavior, Cognition, and Delaying institutionalization. Our general practice is to continue patients on cognitive enhancers as long as at least one of these goals remains, taking into account any issues with costs or adverse effects. Behavior is often a goal of therapy, even in late-stage dementia and sometimes withdrawing drugs such as a cholinesterase inhibitor or NMDA antagonist can unmask or worsen behavioral problems. If the decision has been made to stop one or more medications, we recommend choosing one medication at a time to titrate down (slowly reducing the dose of the medication, similarly to how it was titrated up when it was started). We recommend making only one medication reduction each week, if possible, so that it can easily be re-upped or restarted, if needed. It is generally best not to change more than one neuropsychiatric medication at a time.

In the next chapter, we review alternate therapies, and we discuss medications for mood and behavioral aspects of dementia in subsequent chapters.

Summary

Dementia medications should be started and reduced slowly, but deserve a fair trial at a fair dose. Titration and consistency help reduce potential side effects and may be facilitated through use of a pillbox (or pillboxes) and supervision to ensure medication compliance. Cholinesterase Inhibitors (CIs) are FDA-approved to treat AD. One CI (rivastigmine) is also FDA-approved to treat PDD. Memantine is FDA-approved for the treatment of moderate-to-severe AD. Consider a patient's current symptoms and medical history in choosing dementia medications and the order in which to start them. Treating vascular risk factors constitutes an essential primary or adjunctive treatment of dementia, depending on the type. Regular review of a patient's medication regimen is also well advised.

Common Sense Rules

- All medications have side effects.
- Make medication changes only with a doctor's supervision.
- Use a pillbox and increase supervision as needed.
- Don't start (or stop) more than one medication at a time.
- Don't change medications during major transitions or disruptions to routine.
- Don't stop a dementia medication due to "no change."
- Adjust the timing of a medication to enhance normal sleep–wake cycle.
- Don't switch medications in the same class without good reason.
- Use side effects to a patient's advantage.
- Do not expect dramatic improvements.
- What's good for the heart is good for the brain.

Websites

Alzheimer's Association: Medications for Memory Loss: http://www.alz.org/alzheimers_disease_standard_prescriptions.asp

Mayo Clinic Drugs and Supplements: http://www.mayoclinic.com/health/drug-information/DrugHerbIndex

Medline Plus: http://www.nlm.nih.gov/medlineplus/druginformation.html

References

1. Farlow MR, Boustani M. Pharmacological treatment of Alzheimer disease and mild cognitive impairment. In: Weiner MF, Lipton AM, editors. The American psychiatric publishing textbook of Alzheimer disease and other dementias. Washington, DC: American Psychiatric Publishing, Inc.; 2009.
2. Volicer L, Simard J. Management of advanced dementia. In: Weiner MF, Lipton AM, editors. The American psychiatric publishing textbook of Alzheimer disease and other dementias. Washington, DC: American Psychiatric Publishing, Inc.; 2009.
3. Geldmacher DS, Provenzano G, McRae T, Mastey V, Ieni JR. Donepezil is associated with delayed nursing home placement in patients with Alzheimer's disease. J Am Geriatr Soc. 2003;51(7):937–44.
4. Cappell J, Herrmann N, Cornish S, Lanctôt KL. The pharmacoeconomics of cognitive enhancers in moderate to severe Alzheimer's disease. CNS Drugs. 2010;24(11):909–27. doi:10.2165/11539530-000000000-00000.
5. Wimo A, Winblad B, Stoffler A, Wirth Y, Mobius HJ. Resource utilisation and cost analysis of memantine in patients with moderate to severe Alzheimer's disease. Pharmacoeconomics. 2003;21(5):327–40.
6. Perry EK, Tomlinson BE, Blessed G, Bergmann K, Gibson PH, Perry RH. Correlation of cholinergic abnormalitities with senile plaques and mental test scores in senile dementia. Br Med J. 1978;2(6150):1457–9.
7. Bierer LM, Haroutunian V, Gabriel S, Knott PJ, Carlin LS, Purohit DP, Perl DP, Schmeidler J, Kanof P, Davis KL. Neurochemical correlates of dementia severity in Alzheimer's disease: relative importance of the cholinergic deficits. J Neurochem. 1995;64(2):749–60.
8. Emre M, Aarsland D, Albanese A, et al. Rivastigmine for dementia associated with Parkinson's disease. N Engl J Med. 2004;351:2509–18.
9. Thomas AJ, Burn DJ, Rowan EN, Littlewood E, Newby J, Cousins D, Pakrasi S, Richardson J, Sanders J, McKeith IG. A comparison of the efficacy of donepezil in Parkinson's disease with dementia and dementia with Lewy bodies. Int J Geriatr Psychiatry. 2005;20(10):938–44.
10. Litvinenko IV, Odinak MM, Mogil'naya VI, Emelin AY. Efficacy and safety of galantamine (reminyl) for dementia in patients with Parkinson's disease (an open controlled trial). Neurosci Behav Physiol. 2008;38(9):937–45.
11. Grace J, Amick MM, Friedman JH. A double-blind comparison of galantamine hydrobromide ER and placebo in Parkinson disease. J Neurol Neurosurg Psychiatry. 2009;80(1):18–23. Epub 2008 Oct 17.
12. Abbott RD, Petrovitch H, White LR, et al. Frequency of bowel movements and the future risk of Parkinson's disease. Neurology. 2001;57(3):456–62.
13. Winblad B, Poritis N. Memantine in severe dementia: results of the 9 M-Best Study (Benefit and efficacy in severely demented patients during treatment with memantine). Int J Geriatr Psychiatry. 1999;14(2):135–46.
14. Mobius HJ, Stoffler A. Memantine in vascular dementia. Int Psychogeriatr. 2003;15 Suppl 1:207–13.
15. Orgogozo JM, Rigaud AS, Stoffler A, Mobius HJ, Forette F. Efficacy and safety of memantine in patients with mild to moderate vascular dementia: a randomized, placebo-controlled trial (MMM 300). Stroke. 2002;33(7):1834–9.
16. Kavirajan H, Schneider LS. Efficacy and adverse effects of cholinesterase inhibitors and memantine in vascular dementia: a meta-analysis of randomized controlled trials. Lancet Neurol. 2007;6(9):782–92.
17. Aarsland D, Ballard C, Walker Z, Bostrom F, Alves G, Kossakowski K, Leroi I, Pozo-Rodriguez F, Minthon L, Londos E. Memantine in patients with Parkinson's disease dementia or dementia with Lewy bodies: a double-blind, placebo-controlled, multicentre trial. Lancet Neurol. 2009;8(7):613–8. Epub 2009 Jun 10.

18. Emre M, Tsolaki M, Bonuccelli U, Destée A, Tolosa E, Kutzelnigg A, Ceballos-Baumann A, Zdravkovic S, Bladström A, Jones R, 11018 Study Investigators. Memantine for patients with Parkinson's disease dementia or dementia with Lewy bodies: a randomised, double-blind, placebo-controlled trial. Lancet Neurol. 2010;9(10):969–77. Epub 2010 Aug 20.
19. Boxer A, Womack K, Lipton AM, et al. An open label study of memantine treatment in three subtypes of frontotemporal lobar degeneration. Alzheimer Dis Assoc Disord. 2009;23(3): 211–7.
20. Tariot PN, Farlow MR, Grossberg GT, et al. Memantine treatment in patients with moderate to severe Alzheimer disease already receiving donepezil: a randomized controlled trial. JAMA. 2004;291(3):317–24.
21. Cummings JL, Schneider E, Tariot PN, Graham SM, Memantine MEM-MD-02 Study Group. Behavioral effects of memantine in Alzheimer disease patients receiving donepezil treatment. Neurology. 2006;67(1):57–63.
22. Feldman HH, Schmitt FA, Olin JT, Memantine MEM-MD-02 Study Group. Activities of daily living in moderate-to-severe Alzheimer disease: an analysis of the treatment effects of memantine in patients receiving stable donepezil treatment. Alzheimer Dis Assoc Disord. 2006;20(4):263–8.

Chapter 9
Alternative Therapies in Dementia

"The best doctors in the world are Dr. Diet, Dr. Quiet and Dr. Merryman."

—Jonathan Swift

In this chapter, we discuss nutritional and other nonmedication approaches to dementia. Whether such strategies prevent cognitive impairment in people without preexisting dementia is a worthy topic and we touch on it, but an extensive discussion of therapies for prevention of cognitive impairment in healthy individuals is beyond the scope of this book and chapter. Our discussion instead focuses mainly on patients who already have dementia.

We also limit our discussion to methods that have been studied in dementia and/ or are commonly used by our patients and families, but inclusion does not equal efficacy. In fact, we list several products and procedures that don't help—and may hurt. If we don't mention a supplement that means that it doesn't have enough evidence as of the time of writing this book to be considered for clinical use in dementia (although it may need more study and have a role in research studies in dementia). If you are interested in alternate therapies, we encourage you to consult reliable resources (i.e., not simply relying on the manufacturer and/or seller of a product for information) and certainly consider participation in research studies of promising treatments, to help us all learn more.

Diet

You may have anticipated that we would open this chapter with an introduction to supplements. However, diet is key to this discussion. In reviewing data from nutritional research and cognitive decline, evidence emerges that taking supplements may be the least effective means to a positive end. Furthermore, even when dietary intake

A.M. Lipton and C.D. Marshall, *The Common Sense Guide to Dementia for Clinicians and Caregivers*, DOI 10.1007/978-1-4614-4163-2_9, © Springer Science+Business Media, LLC 2013

is considered, the benefit of one's diet as a whole may be greater than individual dietary factors. For example, vitamin E supplementation does not appear to prevent cognitive decline in normal individuals or patients with Mild Cognitive Impairment (MCI) [1] or AD [2] However, some studies have found that a high dietary intake of vitamin E may help prevent AD [3, 4] and other types of dementia. [5]. Of course, eating a healthy diet requires more attention and effort than does just taking pills.

It should also be noted that much more research has been done on the role of dietary factors in preventing cognitive decline in healthy individuals than in patients who already have dementia. However, a healthy diet may be meaningful not only for primary prevention, but also for treatment (or so-called "secondary prevention") of dementia. The research on overall diet that has been done in patients with dementia has primarily focused on AD. The so-called "Mediterranean Diet" is rich in vegetables, complex carbohydrates, unsaturated fat/olive oil while low in meat products and saturated fat. It also includes regular but moderate alcohol intake (see more about alcohol and dementia in the following chapter). This diet may help not only protect against cognitive decline in healthy individuals but also reduce cognitive decline in MCI [6] and AD [7] as well as reduce mortality in AD [8]. In accordance with the above findings, such a diet would naturally be high in vitamin E.

Recall that what's good for the heart is good for the brain. And, when it comes to nutritional factors, overall diet probably supersedes supplementation.

Common sense rule: It's not the supplements, it's the diet.

The next section of this chapter addresses nutritional and botanical supplements in dementia. Other dietary intake considerations in dementia, including poor appetite and weight loss as the disease progresses, will be discussed in later chapters.

Nutritional and Botanical Supplements in Dementia

For medications to receive FDA approval for efficacy for a particular medical condition, the drugs must be studied in humans as well as animals and shown to be effective in people with the specific medical condition for which they are approved (i.e., have an indication). However, botanical and nutritional supplements (including vitamins, minerals, and food products) are not regulated by the FDA a as medications. What this means is that manufacturers, marketers, and other sellers of nutritional and botanical products can (and do) make questionable claims of efficacy. Such products are also not regulated for purity (so you can't guarantee what you're getting). And, while just like medications, nutritional and botanical remedies carry risks, the FDA does not require the same routine monitoring for adverse events by the manufacturers as it does for pharmaceutical companies.

Common sense rule: Buyer and caregiver, beware.

Like most things in life, if it sounds good to be true, it probably is. If such remedies are to be tried, the following points are important to take into account:

- *Consider Quality of Life.* We have had family caregivers administer upwards of 20 natural and/or nutritional daily (or expect a patient with dementia to self-administer the same). Such a regimen is unrealistic and detrimental to quality of life for caregiver and patient in terms of time, effort, and money spent. It is one thing for a patient to have to take a medication three or more times daily to help them breathe or move, such as may be the case for a patient with COPD or Parkinson's disease, but such supplements are unlikely to impact quality of life in the same way. If such products are to be used, use them selectively, just as you would any medication, because as previously noted.
- *All medications have risks, including alternate therapies.* We recommend checking with a patient's physicians regarding potential benefits, side effects, and interactions of each treatment. Natural does not necessarily mean better.
- *Beware the "magic bullet" phenomenon.* If there was one, we would be very happy to let you and all our patients and families know about it. Many substances have been studied for treating dementia and none is a "magic bullet." In fact, some have been shown to be ineffective in very good clinical studies. And, keeping that all such products have risks, carefully weigh harm versus good, including consideration of the cost of such treatments.
- *Beware the 6 O'Clock News phenomenon.* If the results of a study of any drug sound incredible, retain a healthy skepticism. Find out whether research was done in humans or not. Sometimes studies done in animals or on tissue samples in a petri dish do NOT translate to efficacy for people. Also, sometimes such research may involve directly injecting a medication into brain tissue or an animal's brain. If a vitamin or other supplement is given by mouth to a person, it might be dissolved by acid in the stomach. It might also be too large to cross over the specialized blood–brain barrier and make it into the brain. A clinical study is conducted in living people. A preclinical study is performed on animals, tissue or cells.

Common sense rule: Natural does not necessarily mean better.

Consider the caveats above as you read the following on some specific nutritional and botanical supplements used in dementia, including some that have no good evidence to support their utility in dementia, but they are commonly used nonetheless and/or we are often asked about them.

Vitamins

B Vitamins

Insufficiency of vitamin B12 (cobalamin) can result in anemia, fatigue, depression, and cognitive problems, including memory loss. Since this is one of the few reversible causes of dementia, checking the level of B12 in the blood is part of the routine evaluation for a patient with dementia. Levels of folate (vitamin B9), the amino acid homocysteine, and methylmalonic acid (MMA) may be related to B12 deficiency and may also be checked, along with a complete blood count.

Hyperhomocysteinemia refers to a high level of homocysteine in the blood, may occur along with insufficiency of B12 and/or folate, and increases risks of vascular disease, such as strokes and heart attacks. It is therefore probably not surprising that hyperhomocysteinemia, is also a risk factor for vascular dementia, but what is perhaps somewhat unexpected is that it is also an independent risk factor for AD [9]. Checking the level of MMA may help detect a mild B12 deficiency.

Intramuscular injection of B12 is often used to correct B12 deficiency, especially initially, but chronic treatment with appropriate oral supplementation (including some preparations available by prescription only) is often sufficient to correct folate and B12 deficiencies [10]. Hyperhomocysteinemia can be treated with a combination of B vitamins (including some prescription only supplements) taken by mouth. However, utilizing such preparations to lower normal homocysteine levels has not shown much benefit and can cause significant problems, including, increased vascular complications, such as stroke and heart attack [11]. Thus, it can be harmful to treat people with high doses of B vitamins if there isn't a specific need. Furthermore treatment with B vitamins doesn't prevent or treat dementia without such abnormalities [12]. In summary, in individuals with normal B12, folate, homocysteine, and MMA levels, B vitamins don't help and can hurt. We therefore recommend that only patients with defined B vitamin deficiencies and/or hyperhomocysteinemia should be treated and even then with close medical supervision.

It is important to note that conditions, such as hyperhomocysteinemia and/or deficiency in B12 and/or folate can be hereditary and, if a patient has one or more of these findings, we recommend that his or her blood relatives also have relevant laboratory tests checked to determine if they could have a similar condition.

Vitamin D

Vitamin D has been variably associated with cognitive impairment and dementia [13] and treatment studies are lacking. Given this lack of evidence, we do not recommend vitamin D for the sole treatment of dementia (or prevention thereof). We generally have our patients consult with their general practitioner to have vitamin D checked and for any suggested supplementation.

Vitamin E

A careful review of scientific studies of vitamin E supplementation at any dose failed to show benefit for patients with AD or MCI [13]. Vitamin E did not prove to be beneficial for patients with Mild Cognitive Impairment (MCI) in a large 3-year clinical study [14]. Furthermore, a daily dosage of vitamin E > 400 International

Units may pose significant risks, including stroke [15] and death [16], for all types of patients.

Vitamin E has adverse effects of bleeding and bruising. This is especially concerning for those who also take blood thinners (e.g., warfarin, trade name: Coumadin), aspirin, ginkgo biloba (see below), or non-steroidal anti-inflammatory drugs (NSAIDS), such as ibuprofen.

Supplements

Acetyl-L-Carnitine

We find many patients with dementia use this supplement despite a lack of benefit based on objective data [17]. The only reason we include it in our discussion is to advise that it isn't worthwhile.

Caprylidene/Caprylic Acid (Trade Name: Axona)

You may have heard of the ketogenic diet for treating epilepsy or coconut oil for treating AD. Caprylidene employs a similar idea to treat AD (but doesn't risk severely increased cholesterol and other lipids as is the case for coconut oil—see below). Based on research that has been done which links impaired glucose metabolism and AD [18], caprylidene is designed to provide an alternate energy source for the brain. Caprylidene is a medical food Generally Recognized as Safe (GRAS) by the FDA. Medical foods are not subject to the same FDA standards of efficacy as are medications. As of the time of writing this book, the published scientific evidence for clinical efficacy (showing that the product works in patients) for caprylidene is limited to a study sponsored by the manufacturer [19], which showed modest benefits for patients with AD over 3 months. On the plus side, this was a randomized controlled trial, the highest standard for clinical research. However, further evidence of efficacy has not been forthcoming.

Caprylidene comes in a powder to be mixed with fluid or soft food and taken daily. It shares similar GI risks, such as nausea and diarrhea, with CIs. Thus, it should be avoided in patients sensitive to the GI effects of CIs or with other significant GI medical or surgical history. For other patients, slowly titrating the dose or using half a dose may minimize adverse GI side effects. Abdominal discomfort (dyspepsia) and abdominal gas (flatulence) are also common with caprylidene.

We concur with the manufacturer's recommendation that it be used cautiously in patients at risk for ketoacidosis or who have GI inflammation, metabolic syndrome, or renal syndrome. For those who may be sensitive to milk and soy, it should be noted that caprylidene contains both of these ingredients. Some patients also can't abide the taste. Finally, since caprylidene is a medical food and not a medication, prescription plans generally will not cover the cost.

Choline/Lecithin

Like acetyl-L-carnitine above, we find that many patients with dementia take oral choline supplementation despite lack of efficacy for human brain disease. You may recall from the previous chapter that levels of acetylcholine are low in the brains of patients with AD. The rationale for choline supplementation is therefore to boost these levels. However, dietary forms of choline (including lecithin) do NOT increase (or in any way affect) the levels of different forms of choline in the human brain [20]. Careful analysis of clinical studies showed choline supplementation is not effective in AD or PDD and may only contribute to adverse effects [21]. The evidence for any benefit for choline supplementation is so weak as not to even justify doing a larger study. We make mention of oral choline supplementation because we have seen so many patients with dementia take it, it doesn't help, and it might hurt.

Coconut Oil

Although there are no studies of coconut oil in dementia, some people use it anyway based on a similar rationale to the one explained above for caprylic acid. However, coconut oil is a significant source of saturated fat and can cause significant increases in "bad" cholesterol and triglycerides. Coconut oil is often used in movie theater popcorn and nondairy creamers and the amount of saturated fat that it adds to these items is a major reason that they are such poor dietary choices. Due to the unhealthy saturated fat that coconut oil contains, the FDA, American Dietetic Association, American Heart Association, and Department of Health and Human Services all recommend against consuming large amounts of it. So, coconut oil lacks any proof of benefit for dementia, but compelling data that it is harmful (by leading to cholesterol buildup and plaques in blood vessels predisposing to vascular complications like stroke, heart attacks, and dementia). In this case what's bad for the heart may also be bad for the brain.

CoEnzyme Q10 (CoQ10) (Ubiquinone, Idebenone)

Mitochondria are the power generators of human cells. CoQ10 is necessary for the normal function of mitochondria and is also an antioxidant which may reduce the damage from by-products (such as "free radicals") produced when mitochondria dysfunction, which may occur in the case of brain injury or disease. Dementia is one example of such neurodegenerative disease.

CoQ10 caused significant slowing of decline in ADLs, cognition, and motor function in patients who were diagnosed with Parkinson's Disease without dementia [22]. CoQ10 was associated with slight cognitive and motor benefit in Progressive Supranuclear Palsy (PSP) [23]. Idebenone, a synthetic form of CoQ10, did not show benefit in a carefully done study of patients with AD [24]. CoQ10 was not found to be beneficial in Amyotrophic Lateral Sclerosis (ALS), including on a mental quality of life measure [25] (we mention this since, as you may recall from Chap. 2, Frontotemporal Dementia (FTD) and ALS may be associated in given patients or families).

CoQ10 possesses a variety of potential adverse effects, including gastrointestinal symptoms, and drug interactions. We therefore recommend checking with a patient's physician before trying any form of CoQ10 and only using it with medical supervision.

Fish Oil/Omega-3 Fatty Acids/DHA

Fish serves as an important dietary source of docosahexanoic acid (DHA), an important brain fatty acid. DHA has been found to be lower in patients with AD than people of the same age with normal memory [26] but DHA supplements do not appear to help patients with AD [27]. A recent large study also showed that dietary fish intake does not appear to prevent dementia of any type [28]. Use of these supplements may be associated with diarrhea. The preponderance of the evidence for fatty acids is insufficient to recommend them as a treatment (or preventive measure) for dementia.

Ginkgo Biloba

Ginkgo biloba is a plant extract widely used for cognitive impairment and dementia. Studies of ginkgo biloba in the treatment of dementia have yielded variable results. However, some evidence supports modest effects of ginkgo biloba in the treatment of dementia. These include modest cognitive benefits for AD, Vascular dementia, and Mixed (AD + Vascular) dementia and modest benefits for ADLs in AD [29]. A dose of 240 mg daily may be required to achieve such benefits. (Ginkgo biloba is often administered in divided daily doses, so a dose of 240 mg daily might be achieved by taking 80 mg three times daily.) Further study of gingko biloba in the treatment of dementia may be helpful. Ginkgo biloba did not prevent AD or other types of dementia based on a careful, large scientific study funded by the National Institute of Health [30].

Huperzine A

Huperzine A is a Chinese herbal remedy touted as a possible cheaper natural alternative to CIs. However, it does not provide benefit over a placebo (sugar pill) in AD [31] and there is no evidence for benefit in other types of dementia. Huperzine A could be harmful to use in conjunction with any CI due to similar side effect profiles. If you are looking for a natural remedy, consider the CI galantamine, which is derived from a flower, the snowdrop, but steer clear of Huperzine A.

Melatonin

Melatonin is secreted as a hormone by the brain's pineal gland in humans and is also found in some plants. Our clinical experience has been that melatonin continues to be widely used to treat dementia symptoms, but there is no evidence to support such use. Melatonin does not benefit behavior, functioning, or cognition in people with dementia. A careful scientific study of melatonin in patients with AD did not show any benefit for sleep or agitation [32].

Phosphatidylserine

This is a component of cell membranes. There is no evidence that this benefits patients who have dementia. Beware marketers who may cite old research with phosphatidylserine from cattle suggested benefit for preventing cognitive impairment. This form is no longer available due to theoretical concerns regarding transmission of bovine spongiform encephalopathy ("mad cow disease"). Research done on soy-derived phosphatidylserine has shown no benefit for prevention or treatment of dementia [33].

Tramiprosate ("Vivimind")

This is marketed as a medical food and is a modification of the amino acid taurine, which is found in seaweed. (An amino acid is a building block of proteins.) It has been studied in patients with AD but had no clear benefit, nor has it been shown to be beneficial in other types of dementia [34].

Common sense rule: Weigh the benefits and risks of supplements.

Stimulatory Therapies

A variety of studies have shown that exercise, socialization, and other activities may benefit quality of life for patients with dementia. Many of these modalities were discussed in Chap. 6 and further information is available in Chap. 13. We recommend tailoring activities to the patient's history, interest, and abilities and continuing activities that a patient enjoys to the degree possible. Enrollment in an adult day program ("brain therapy") may also help by giving the caregiver a break and this is described in depth in Chap. 15: Selecting Level of Care.

Scheduled Voiding

Scheduled voiding has been shown to be efficacious in treating urinary incontinence as previously referenced in Chap. 6.

Other Alternative Therapies

Chelation Therapy

Chelation therapy refers to methods used to eliminate heavy metals. There is no evidence that chelation therapy works for AD [35] or any dementia other than one that is directly attributable to accumulation of heavy metals, such as Wilson's disease (which is associated with buildup of copper) or some types of porphyria associated with increased iron accumulation. Wilson's disease and some cases of porphyria may call for oral and/or intravenous (IV) chelation, but, in other types of dementia, there is no accumulation of any heavy metals and therefore nothing to "chelate." Unscrupulous practitioners may offer expensive, invasive, and worthless IV chelation for the treatment of dementia not due to Wilson's disease or porphyria. Placement of an IV line and associated infusion can be painful and anxiety-provoking for patients. Consequently, except for the rare dementia due to build up of specific heavy metals, avoid intravenous chelation at all costs (financial and otherwise)!

Quantitative Electroencephalogram

The role of EEG in dementia is purely diagnostic and is not always required. Quantitative or any other type of EEG has no therapeutic effect. However, we are aware of families going to great expense and trouble to have quantitative electroencephalogram (qEEG) performed (based on claims made by an unscrupulous provider that it might help the dementia). Although such procedures aren't typically invasive, they may be difficult, especially for patients with advanced dementia, as a patient must remain still for placement of and recording from a number of scalp electrodes.

An EEG may be helpful in some cases for diagnosis, especially to evaluate for seizure or seizures/epilepsy, encephalopathy, or certain types of dementia (Creutzfeldt–Jakob disease). A physician ordering an EEG for diagnostic purposes should be able to explain to you as a caregiver the reason/s for such test. In cases of advanced dementia in which you may be making medical decisions for a patient, you may wish to have a discussion with the doctor as to whether the EEG is necessary. For example, if a patient with advanced dementia has a condition which will not be treated even if found on EEG, it is not necessary to do the EEG. In other words, only do the test if it has the potential to change the plan of care for a patient.

Stem Cell Therapy

There is no evidence that stem cell therapy helps dementia, and it has a host of possible problems. If stem cells are directly implanted in the brain, this obviously involves neurosurgery and its potential complications. Also, the brain is complex and dementia involves widespread problems with brain cells and connections. There is currently no way to get stem cells everywhere they need to go and function in the ways needed. If stem cell therapy is offered via any other route than direct brain implantation, they will not enter the brain as any cell is too large to penetrate the blood–brain barrier. Without regulations such as are followed in the US, pooled and/ or infected stem cells could be injected (and have for some people, resulting in death in some cases [36]). Even with appropriate protections and a carefully done trial, stem cell therapies may have unintended consequences, including worsening of symptoms, such as was the case for a US study of stem cell therapy in patients with Parkinson's disease [37]. Sometimes, the "cure" really can be worse than the disease.

Despite all of these concerns, rogue doctors and/or clinics outside the United States may offer stem cell therapy for dementia—at a steep price. Such treatment would be illegal in the United States outside the auspices of a research study which would not incur a cost for participation. If stem cell therapy remains something of interest, look for a research study (either in the US or someplace with similar safeguards for human subjects) accepting participants free of charge.

We don't recommend transporting a patient with advanced dementia to another country for any type of treatment as the risks of such travel outweigh any benefit.

Common sense rule: Check with a trusted doctor or other medical source.

What Can I Do to Prevent Dementia in Myself?

Although the thrust of this chapter is the role of alternate therapy in dementia, we close with one of the most common questions that we encounter in the clinic. A recent blue-ribbon panel found insufficient evidence to support modifiable risk factors to prevent AD [38]. With that caveat in mind, however, they did find that diabetes mellitus, high cholesterol, and smoking were associated with an increased risk of AD. A similarly qualified reduced risk of AD was found for Mediterranean-type diet, folic acid intake, low or moderate alcohol intake, cognitive activities, and physical activity. Such factors may be even more highly associated with an increased or decreased risk of vascular and mixed (Alzheimer + Vascular) dementia. We recommend that our patients and families follow the common sense rules and activities in Table 9.1 that may enhance quality as well as quantity of life:

Common sense rule: What's good for the heart is good for the brain.

Summary

A heart-healthy diet may present a worthwhile intervention and possible preventive measure for dementia. B vitamin supplementation may be beneficial when a deficiency is detected, but may be contraindicated in the face of normal laboratory

Table 9.1 Measures that may help prevent dementia

• Control vascular risk factors to the extent possible
– Including: diabetes mellitus, cholesterol, triglycerides
– May be worthwhile to have B12/folate and associated markers checked
– Proper dental care and hygiene
• Exercise
• Don't smoke
• Eat a healthy diet rich in vegetables and grains and low in meat and saturated fats
• Engage in social and mental activities that you enjoy (don't force yourself to do things that you don't like—stress and frustration are bad for the brain)
• Treat depression (which is a risk factor for dementia and cardiovascular disease)
• Consider having vitamin D level checked

findings. Insufficient evidence exists to support medical recommendations for other supplements in dementia. Chelation therapy is recommended only for disease states involving accumulation of heavy metals, such as Wilson's disease and some types of porphyria. EEG may be a useful tool for the diagnosis (but not the treatment) of cognitive impairment. Stem cell therapy needs much more research and refinement before it can be considered for clinical treatment of dementia.

Common Sense Rules

- It's not the supplements, it's the diet.
- Natural does not necessarily mean better.
- Buyer and caregiver, beware.
- Weigh the benefits and risks of supplements.
- Check with a trusted doctor or other medical source.
- Don't hang your hat on one thing.
- What's good for the heart is good for the brain.

Websites

Alzheimer's Association: www.alz.org
    National Center for Complementary and Alternative Medicine, National Institutes of Health: www.nccam.nih.gov

References

1. Petersen RC, Thomas RG, Grundman M, et al. Vitamin E and donepezil for the treatment of mild cognitive impairment. N Engl J Med. 2005;352(23):2379–88.
2. Sano M, Ernesto C, Thomas RG, et al. A controlled trial of selegiline, alpha-tocopherol, or both as treatment for Alzheimer's disease. The Alzheimer's Disease Cooperative Study. N Engl J Med. 1997;336(17):1216–22.

3. Engelhart MJ, Geerlings MI, Ruitenberg A, van Swieten JC, Hofman A, Witteman JC, Breteler MM. Dietary intake of antioxidants and risk of Alzheimer disease. JAMA. 2002;287(24): 3223–9.
4. Morris MC, Evans DA, Bienias JL, et al. Dietary intake of antioxidant nutrients and the risk of incident Alzheimer disease in a biracial community study. JAMA. 2002;287(24):3230–7.
5. Devore EE, Grodstein F, van Rooij FJ, Hofman A, Stampfer MJ, Witteman JC, Breteler MM. Dietary antioxidants and long-term risk of dementia. Arch Neurol. 2010;67(7):819–25.
6. Scarmeas N, Stern Y, Mayeux R, Manly JJ, Schupf N, Luchsinger JA. Mediterranean diet and mild cognitive impairment. Arch Neurol. 2009;66(2):216–25.
7. Féart C, Samieri C, Rondeau V, Amieva H, Portet F, Dartigues JF, Scarmeas N, Barberger-Gateau P. Adherence to a Mediterranean diet, cognitive decline, and risk of dementia. JAMA. 2009;302(6):638–48.
8. Scarmeas N, Luchsinger JA, Mayeux R, Stern Y. Mediterranean diet and Alzheimer disease mortality. Neurology. 2007;69(11):1084–93.
9. Seshadri S, Beiser A, Selhub J, Jacques PF, Rosenberg IH, D'Agostino RB, Wilson PW, Wolf PA. Plasma homocysteine as a risk factor for dementia and Alzheimer's disease. N Engl J Med. 2002;346(7):476–83.
10. Kuzminski AM, Del Giacco EJ, Allen RH, Stabler SP, Lindenbaum J. Effective treatment of cobalamin deficiency with oral cobalamin. Blood. 1998;92:1191–8.
11. House A, Eliasziw M. Effect of B-vitamin therapy on progression of diabetic nephropathy. JAMA. 2010;303(16):1603–9.
12. Joosten E. Homocysteine, vascular dementia and Alzheimer's disease. Clin Chem Lab Med. 2001;39(8):717–20.
13. Buell JS, Tucker KL. The value of physiologic vitamin D as a biomarker of dementia. Drugs Today (Barc). 2011;47(3):223–31.
14. Isaac MG, Quinn R, Tabet N. Vitamin E for Alzheimer's disease and mild cognitive impairment. Cochrane Database Syst Rev. 2008;3:CD002854.
15. The Alpha-Tocopherol, Beta Carotene Cancer Prevention Study Group. The effect of vitamin E and beta carotene on the incidence of lung cancer and other cancers in male smokers. N Engl J Med. 1994;330:1029–35.
16. Miller III ER, Pastor-Barriuso R, Dalal D, Riemersma RA, Appel LJ, Guallar E. Meta-analysis: high-dosage vitamin E supplementation may increase all-cause mortality. Ann Intern Med. 2005;142:37–46.
17. Hudson SA, Tabet N. Acetyl-L-carnitine for dementia. Cochrane Database Syst Rev. 2003;2:CD003158. doi:10.1002/14651858.CD003158.
18. Liu F, Shi J, Tanimukai H, Gu J, Gu J, Grundke-Iqbal I, Iqbal K, Gong CX. Reduced O-GlcNAcylation links lower brain glucose metabolism and tau pathology in Alzheimer's disease. Brain. 2009;132(Pt 7):1820–32. Epub 2009 May 18.
19. Henderson ST, Vogel JL, Barr LJ, Garvin F, Jones JJ, Costantini LC. Study of the ketogenic agent AC-1202 in mild to moderate Alzheimer's disease: a randomized, double-blind, placebo-controlled, multicenter trial. Nutr Metab. 2009;6:31.
20. Higgins JPT, Flicker L. Lecithin for dementia and cognitive impairment. Cochrane Database Syst Rev. 2000;4:CD001015. doi:10.1002/14651858.CD001015.
21. Tan J, Bluml S, Hoang T, Dubowitz D, Mevenkamp G, Ross B. Lack of effect of oral choline supplement on the concentrations of choline metabolites in human brain. Magn Reson Med. 1998;39(6):1005–10.
22. Shults CW, Oakes D, Kieburtz K, Beal MF, Haas R, Plumb S, Juncos JL, Nutt J, Shoulson I, Carter J, Kompoliti K, Perlmutter JS, Reich S, Stern M, Watts RL, Kurlan R, Molho E, Harrison M, Lew M, Parkinson Study Group. Effects of coenzyme Q10 in early Parkinson disease: evidence of slowing of the functional decline. Arch Neurol. 2002;59(10):1541–50.
23. Stamelou M, Reuss A, Pilatus U, Magerkurth J, Niklowitz P, Eggert KM, Krisp A, Menke T, Schade-Brittinger C, Oertel WH, Höglinger GU. Short-term effects of coenzyme Q10 in progressive supranuclear palsy: a randomized, placebo-controlled trial. Mov Disord. 2008;23(7): 942–9.

24. Thal LJ, Grundman M, Berg J, Ernstrom K, Margolin R, Pfeiffer E, Weiner MF, Zamrini E, Thomas RG. Idebenone treatment fails to slow cognitive decline in Alzheimer's disease. Neurology. 2003;61(11):1498–502.

25. Kaufmann P, Thompson JL, Levy G, Buchsbaum R, Shefner J, Krivickas LS, Katz J, Rollins Y, Barohn RJ, Jackson CE, Tiryaki E, Lomen-Hoerth C, Armon C, Tandan R, Rudnicki SA, Rezania K, Sufit R, Pestronk A, Novella SP, Heiman-Patterson T, Kasarskis EJ, Pioro EP, Montes J, Arbing R, Vecchio D, Barsdorf A, Mitsumoto H, Levin B, QALS Study Group. Phase II trial of CoQ10 for ALS finds insufficient evidence to justify phase III. Ann Neurol. 2009;66(2):235–44.

26. Conquer JA, Tierney MC, Zecevic J, Bettger WJ, Fisher RH. Fatty acid analysis of blood plasma of patients with Alzheimer's disease, other types of dementia, and cognitive impairment. Lipids. 2000;35(12):1305–12.

27. Quinn JF, Raman R, Thomas RG, Yurko-Mauro K, Nelson EB, Van Dyck C, Galvin JE, Emond J, Jack Jr CR, Weiner M, Shinto L, Aisen PS. Docosahexaenoic acid supplementation and cognitive decline in Alzheimer disease: a randomized trial. JAMA. 2010;304(17):1903–11.

28. Devore EE, Grodstein F, van Rooij FJ, Hofman A, Rosner B, Stampfer MJ, Witteman JC, Breteler MM. Dietary intake of fish and omega-3 fatty acids in relation to long-term dementia risk. Am J Clin Nutr. 2009;90(1):170–6. Epub 2009 May 27.

29. Weinmann S, Roll S, Schwarzbach C, Vauth C, Willich SN. Effects of Ginkgo biloba in dementia: systematic review and meta-analysis. BMC Geriatr. 2010;10:14.

30. DeKosky ST, Williamson JD, Fitzpatrick AL, Kronmal RA, Ives DG, Saxton JA. Ginkgo biloba for prevention of dementia: a randomized controlled trial. JAMA. 2008;300:2253–62. doi:10.1001/jama.2008.683.

31. Rafii MS, Walsh S, Little JT, Behan K, Reynolds B, Ward C, Jin S, Thomas R, Aisen PS, Alzheimer's Disease Cooperative Study. A phase II trial of huperzine A in mild to moderate Alzheimer disease. Neurology. 2011;76(16):1389–94.

32. Gehrman PR, Connor DJ, Martin JL, Shochat T, Corey-Bloom J, Ancoli-Israel S. Melatonin fails to improve sleep or agitation in double-blind randomized placebo-controlled trial of institutionalized patients with Alzheimer disease. Am J Geriatr Psychiatry. 2009;17(2):166–9.

33. Wollen KA. Alzheimer's disease: the pros and cons of pharmaceutical, nutritional, botanical, and stimulatory therapies, with a discussion of treatment strategies from the perspective of patients and practitioners. Altern Med Rev. 2010;15(3):223–44.

34. Sabbagh MN. Drug development for Alzheimer's disease: where are we now and where are we headed? Am J Geriatr Pharmacother. 2009;7(3):167–85.

35. Cardelli MB, Russell M, Bagne CA, Pomara N. Chelation therapy. Unproved modality in the treatment of Alzheimer-type dementia. J Am Geriatr Soc. 1985;33(8):548–51.

36. Tuffs A. Stem cell treatment in Germany is under scrutiny after child's death. BMJ. 2010;341:c6203. doi:10.1136/bmj.c6203.

37. Olanow CW, Goetz CG, Kordower JH, Stoessl AJ, Sossi V, Brin MF, Shannon KM, Nauert GM, Perl DP, Godbold J, Freeman TB. A double-blind controlled trial of bilateral fetal nigral transplantation in Parkinson's disease. Ann Neurol. 2003;54(3):403–14.

38. Daviglus ML, Plassman BL, Pirzada A, Bell CC, Bowen PE, Burke JR, Connolly Jr ES, Dunbar-Jacob JM, Granieri EC, McGarry K, Patel D, Trevisan M, Williams Jr JW. Risk factors and preventive interventions for Alzheimer disease: state of the science. Arch Neurol. 2011;68(9):1185–90. Epub 2011 May 9.

Chapter 10
Alcohol and Other Substances

Be a victor of your good judgment and not a victim of your bad.

The good news is that light-to-moderate alcohol use does not appear to increase one's risk of dementia In fact, a review of over a hundred studies looking at the relationship of alcohol to cognition found that light to moderate alcohol use, particularly wine, reduces the risk of both Alzheimer's and vascular dementia [1]. Moderate alcohol consumption is typically defined as no more than one drink a day for women or no more than two drinks a day for men. Acknowledging some amount of variation, a drink is typically defined as 12 ounces of beer, 5 ounces of wine, or 1.5 ounces of liquor. The same review [1] found that heavy drinking was associated with an increased risk of dementia.

It is important to note that these studies looked at the effects of drinking on the cognition of nondemented individuals. Once a dementia diagnosis is in place, we must consider other relevant factors. When combined with age and/or dementia, alcohol, even in low-to-moderate amounts has diverse potential hazards. Alcohol use increases the risks of depression, disinhibition, confusion, and falls for an older person and/or one with dementia. Therefore, a patient with dementia shouldn't start drinking alcohol or more alcohol than he or she did prior to their dementia diagnosis. In fact, since the brain of a patient with dementia is often exquisitely vulnerable to the amnestic effects of alcohol, we often recommend reducing or even ceasing alcohol intake (with medical supervision) once a diagnosis of dementia is made. Such changes should be made with medical supervision and conducted slowly in the case of substantial alcohol intake as abrupt discontinuation can cause serious withdrawal effects, including seizures and death.

Common sense rules:

- Dementia may increase the effects of alcohol.
- Alcohol withdrawal should be a gradual, supervised process.

A.M. Lipton and C.D. Marshall, *The Common Sense Guide to Dementia for Clinicians and Caregivers*, DOI 10.1007/978-1-4614-4163-2_10, © Springer Science+Business Media, LLC 2013

It is imperative to honestly inform a patient's physician of alcohol intake and any associated issues. In our experience, it is not unusual for patients to minimize or omit alcohol use when providing their medical history. In the outpatient setting, primary care physicians may prescribe sedatives (such as sleeping pills) or other medication which may interact with alcohol.

The consequences of an uninformed medical team are even greater in a hospital setting. An inpatient admission may be an abrupt introduction to sobriety for a patient with alcohol dependence. After a few days, signs of alcohol withdrawal may emerge, such as unstable vital signs (e.g., tachycardia, which is an increased heart rate), altered mental status, delirium tremens ("DTs," tremor, or "shakes"), or even seizures. Likewise, we may see an alcohol withdrawal syndrome after a planned or emergent surgery.

No matter how intelligent and educated your doctor is, alcohol withdrawal is not typically at the top of the differential diagnosis (list of possible diagnoses) for elderly patients with dementia who develop changes in their mental status. A physician's lack of awareness of significant alcohol intake could lead to severe consequences for a patient, including death or disability (e.g., brain injury due to unanticipated seizures or other neurological consequences of sudden alcohol withdrawal). The patient might also be unnecessarily subjected to futile testing or treatment, with attendant costs and other risks, in a search for other possibilities. The good news is that informed hospital medical staff can forego these unnecessary options and proactively utilize medications to avert withdrawal symptoms in your loved one. Therefore, please alert medical personnel regarding alcohol use on or before a patient's admission to a hospital or surgery clinic. As discussed in Chaps. 4 and 5, it may help keep the peace to put such sensitive information in writing and convey it discreetly.

Common sense rule: A patient's physician must be informed of alcohol intake.

How much alcohol is too much? The answer is highly individualized and depends on a given patient and circumstances. And, just as is the case for medications, alcohol intake and associated factors should be regularly reassessed by a physician and other caregivers. If alcohol use repeatedly causes problems, then it is probably too much. If Mom has dementia, but is doing well and enjoying her usual glass of wine with dinner, there may be no need to intervene. It is another story if Mom has an occasional glass of wine and begins to hallucinate every time she does so. Or, if she starts with a glass of wine at dinner and then drinks herself into a stupor (perhaps forgetting, maybe even more than once in an evening, that she has already had her usual glass of wine—or more).

Common sense rule: Patients with dementia can overdo alcohol due to forgetfulness, dependence, and/or other factors.

If the issue is merely forgetfulness, then alcohol in a moderate quantity might be administered and supervised by a caregiver, if it is important for a patient's quality of life. On the other hand, since alcohol may be contributing to such memory loss, a patient might be better off without it, especially if it won't be missed. Sometimes a nonalcoholic beverage can be substituted without much fanfare. The best solution is usually to work in concert with medical supervision, weighing the risks and benefits for an individual patient.

Common sense rule: Regularly review the risks and benefits of alcohol for a person with dementia.

Common Sense Approach to Alcohol Dependence in Dementia

Let's say that alcohol is a problem for a loved one with dementia beyond just forgetting. In other words, he or she is knowingly and regularly drinking alcohol to excess. This is typically either a longstanding problem or an exacerbation of one. As noted above, it is a crucial issue to raise with the patient's doctor. What are the options in such a case? Medicare and/or other insurance programs may cover short-term inpatient detoxification, typically in a psychiatric unit. However, such coverage for outpatient substance abuse programs is limited. Outpatient substance abuse programs utilize educational tools, so a patient must have good memory and other cognitive functioning to benefit. One must also be able to engage in introspection to benefit from psychotherapy. Thus, from a practical standpoint, it is rare that a cognitively impaired individual would benefit from a formal alcohol treatment program.

We must also acknowledge similar limitations in trying to convince a loved one not to drink. This is an ineffective strategy in the cognitively intact individual who drinks in excess, so we are not going to pursue such a course for an individual with dementia. Instead, we recommend a practical approach to reducing problematic alcohol consumption.

If a patient can make his or her own decisions, then he or she must be involved in the medical plan of care. If a patient is no longer able to make medical decisions, the person with Medical Power of Attorney must be involved. Family dynamics, particularly within a family dealing with alcoholism, can be complicated. For example, we sometimes learn that a family member is supplying the alcohol for the cognitively impaired individual. Although a patient with dementia and alcohol dependence may lack the introspection necessary for successful psychotherapy, a psychiatrist or other therapist knowledgeable in addiction issues may be helpful for the family.

Common sense rule: Psychotherapy doesn't usually work for patients with significant dementia, but may help family caregivers.

Abrupt discontinuation of alcohol should be avoided due to risk of serious withdrawal symptoms, including seizures and death. Instead a slow taper as directed by a doctor is recommended. However, it is not just medical supervision that is important in this process. Monitoring, supervision, or even greater involvement by a family member is often crucial in helping a patient with dementia stop drinking. A family should work with a patient's doctors, particularly a psychiatrist or other dementia specialist, as to the best strategy. Techniques may include diluting the alcohol with water or other nonalcoholic beverage. Another strategy is to switch to non-alcoholic beer and wine. If a patient is unable to make his or her own medical decisions and a doctor recommends that a family caregiver makes such substitutions, it is usually best to do so in a subtle and circumspect manner, just as you would in making any changes in the daily routine of a loved one with severe dementia.

Common sense rules:

- Alcohol cessation should be a gradual, supervised process (this bears repeating).
- Maintain a daily routine for the person with dementia.

Potential Prescription Drugs of Abuse in Dementia

Apropos of daily routine, good sleep hygiene represents a key component for everyone, including patients with dementia and their caregivers. Unfortunately, disruption of the sleep–wake cycle arises commonly in dementia. Studies indicate that sleep disturbance occurs in around a half to three-quarters of Alzheimer's patients [2, 3]. Sometimes such problems may be satisfactorily addressed with behavioral and environmental measures such as instituting or reinforcing regular bedtimes and wake-up times (see Chap. 13 for additional suggestions). Reviewing and adjusting medication, particularly the timing of administration, may help (see Chap. 8 for further details regarding these approaches). Some patients may benefit from a sleep study, particularly if Obstructive Sleep Apnea (OSA) is suspected due to significant snoring or periods of interrupted breathing during sleep. However, sometimes the addition of a medication (which may be referred to as a sleeping pill, sedative, or sleep aid) may be necessary to treat insomnia effectively.

In this section, we discuss the two classes of prescription medication that we have observed most often used to excess by patients with dementia: Opiates and Sedatives (including benzodiazepines).

Opiates are narcotic medications commonly prescribed for the treatment of severe pain. Examples include codeine and morphine. Under no circumstance do we recommend withholding adequate medication for acute or chronic pain syndromes. In fact, treating pain sufficiently may prevent and/or reduce agitation, irritability, depression, and similar symptoms in dementia. We therefore fully support their use when medically warranted. However, patients can become dependent on opiates, resulting in overutilization, which is the focus of this section.

Common sense rules:

- Good sleep hygiene and pain management may alleviate some dementia symptoms.
- Even prescription drugs may be overutilized.

A sedative is a medication that makes a person sleepy. All sleeping pills, including benzodiazepines, are sedatives, by definition. Opiates can also be sedating. Sleeping pills are generally taken before bedtime for insomnia, although some patients use them if they awaken during the night. We generally recommend that patients do not take such medications after midnight due to the residual morning grogginess that may result. Many other medications prescribed for many other reasons may have a side effect of sedation to which elderly patients may be especially vulnerable. Sometimes alcohol is used as a sleeping aid, but we don't recommend this, as alcohol actually reduces the amount of deep, dreaming sleep.

Benzodiazepines are a class of drugs commonly prescribed to treat anxiety and/or insomnia. They are also used to treat seizures (epilepsy). Although the term benzodiazepine may be unfamiliar, this category of medications includes commonly prescribed drugs such as alprazolam (trade name: Xanax), clonazepam (trade name: Klonopin), diazepam (trade name: Valium), lorazepam (trade name: Ativan), and temazepam (trade name: Restoril). As you can see, a medication with a scientific (generic) name ending in a suffix of -lam or -pam may be a benzodiazepine and, therefore, a sedative (as always, check with a patient's doctor and/or pharmacist, if you're not sure).

However, sometimes the calming effects of these medications lead a patient to use them in managing internal states of unrest, discomfort, or angst that accompanies memory loss. This is another common way people get into trouble with these medications. So, if your loved one with dementia is struggling, he or she may take sedatives or pain medication at regular intervals to get through the day. It is important to consider anxiety as a potential driving force for regular use of "as needed" medications. When patients are in distress, they reach for medications that will settle their mind and body. So if we want to identify underlying anxiety it can be addressed with both environmental intervention and medication that has minimal negative cognitive effects. This is discussed in greater detail in Part 3.

Common sense rules: Use sedating medications cautiously.

Opiates, benzodiazepines, and other classes of medication can cause disinhibition and confusion, particularly in elderly patients and those with dementia. Be mindful that your family member may not include these medications on a medication list due to taking them "as needed" rather than as a "standing dose" (e.g., twice daily at regular times and intervals). It is not unusual for us to learn during a painstaking medical history-taking process that, in addition to the drugs included on the medication listed provided to us, a new patient also takes a sedative a couple times a day along or a sleeping pill at night—or both. It is much better and easier to have this information up front.

  Sedatives have a withdrawal syndrome similar to alcohol and any discontinuation should likewise be gradual. Such gradual withdrawal with medical supervision is a good rule to follow for any substance that affects the brain, especially for geriatric patients. This includes opiates, which have their own withdrawal syndrome. Just as we "start low and go slow" with neuropsychiatric medications, particularly in the elderly, it is also prudent to taper off slowly.

Common sense rule: Medication withdrawal should be a gradual, supervised process.

Keep in mind that a patient may see a primary care physician and multiple specialists. Unfortunately, this creates opportunities for miscommunication and duplication of medication. For example, Dad may receive a prescription for a "nerve pill" (sedative) from his cardiologist and one for a sleeping pill (another sedative) from his family doctor. Although specialists typically communicate with the referring or primary physician, it is quite possible that not all of a patient's physicians communicate with one another or that every prescription change is relayed even to a patient's general practitioner. Therefore, a wise caregiver keeps track of medications and helps keep a patient's physicians informed of these as well (which may be easily done by maintaining an accurate and up-to-date medication list). In addition to the challenges of fragmented communication, Dad's memory issues may impair his ability to keep an accurate medication list and/or report pertinent changes to his physicians. This leads to risk of physician overprescribing or medication duplication.

Common sense rule: A medication list helps avoid drug duplication.

As is the case for alcohol, several common factors can lead to overuse of medication in dementia, especially opiates and sedatives. Any patient (with or without dementia) may become dependent on opiates and/or sedatives. However, patients with dementia may use opiates, sedatives, and/or other medications to excess purely due to forgetfulness. Some patients who have previously used opiates and sedatives to manage specific pain, anxiety and sleep problems may begin to use them to treat other uncomfortable psychological states that can accompany dementia. In addition, a patient may be unknowingly prescribed duplicate or similar medication.

Overutilization can apply to any medication. The only way to know for sure is to monitor the situation. Check to see if your loved one has gone off course and is taking medication more times a day than prescribed. You can view the physician's original instructions by reading the prescription bottle label. You can check the date and amount supplied, the amount to be taken daily, and count any remaining pills to see if a patient seems to be taking too many or not enough.

Never underestimate how even mild memory loss can greatly impair one's ability to take medication correctly. In addition to remembering to take the medication on schedule, a patient has to remember which drugs have already been taken each day to avoid double- or greater overdosing. A weekly pillbox may help diminish this possibility (see also Chap. 6). When in doubt, a patient can check the pillbox to help recall whether or not medications were taken. However, this strategy doesn't work for someone with dementia who can't remember what day of the week it is! Such an individual needs more help and supervision than merely filling a weekly pillbox with. A reminder phone call may be effective for some. Alarmed pillboxes/dispensers are often too complicated and novel for our patients with dementia to learn to use. Unfortunately, a problem with sedatives and opiates is that they may be prescribed on a PRN or "as needed" basis and are therefore not included in a patient's pillbox. For example, a patient might keep a bottle of sleeping pills on the nightstand for convenience. Or, a patient may react to each individual symptom by taking medications instead of sticking with a prescribed treatment plan. In such cases, it may be helpful to instead use a separate pillbox just for the PRN/ as needed medications—and perhaps putting this on the nightstand instead of the entire bottle.

Common sense rules:

- Memory functioning is critical for correct medication administration.
- Monitor medication administration and increase supervision as needed.

Bowel Products

It is not uncommon for our geriatric patients to obsess over their bowels, expecting at least one "movement" a day, and considering anything short of that as pathological. Unfortunately, we also commonly see misuse or abuse of medications such as antidiarrheals, laxatives, and/or stool softeners adversely impacting quality of life. Such overutilization may reflect longstanding habits. It might also represent new behavior (or exacerbation of an old practice) due to the effects of medication and/or cognitive impairment, especially an underlying disturbance in memory and/or executive functioning (such as judgment and problem-solving).

A vicious cycle may commence in which a patient self-administers an antidiarrheal medication after an episode of diarrhea, then becomes constipated and take a stool softener and/or laxative. Depending on the patient's level of cognitive impairment and other psychological issues, he or she may continue to chase after each symptom (diarrhea or constipation) and lose sight of the big picture. Such repetitious and circular use of these remedies may create dependence on such medications, impede resumption of normal gastrointestinal (GI) functioning, and compound GI side effects of other illnesses and medications.

Monitoring the bowel regimen of a loved one who is elderly and/or has dementia may be exceedingly beneficial. Geriatric patients often have bowel problems and concerns. Cognitive and behavioral problems may result in overusage and the drug cascade noted above. And, of particular note, prescription medications for dementia may also affect GI functioning. Mere reliance on someone's report of their bowel regimen may not be enough, particularly if he or she has memory loss for recent events or a vested interest in protecting lifestyle habits. You may need to verify the information provided. If you live with your loved one with dementia, it may facilitate determination of bowel frequency. If you don't, you might stay with them for a few days (including overnight) and try to obtain a fuller picture. Of course, you could have your relative stay with you, but an individual's usual environment and routine, including diet and exercise, typically provides more accurate information. If your relative is in a supervised living situation, you may be able to have nursing staff record this information (a doctor's order may be required). (A week or two of such notation may suffice for this purpose unless any problems emerge).

If you are a primary caregiver, know and review all medications (including those kept in kitchen, bedroom, or bathroom drawers, medication chests, pillboxes, cabinets, etc.), especially in response to any new GI issue. Remember that even patients living in supervised communities may be purchasing laxatives and the like over-the-counter.

Bowel frequency (how often a patient has bowel movements) varies for individuals based on a number of factors. If a patient is having a bowel movement at least every other day, this is quite likely sufficient. If your loved one is not having bowel movements at least every other day, check with a patient's doctor. Less often may call for dietary or medical intervention as might other significant and persistent changes in bowel frequency (e.g., someone who used to have 1–2 bowel movements daily and now has 5 every day).

Once again, diet and exercise are cornerstones of treatment and prevention. A patient's doctor may recommend encouraging hydration, high-fiber foods (including eating fruits and vegetables rather than drinking juice which contains little fiber), fiber and similar supplements, exercise, and medications (over-the-counter and/or prescription),where indicated. Sometimes patients with dementia forget to eat or drink. Therefore, you may wish to place appropriate food and beverage in plain sight (rather than behind the opaque refrigerator door where it may be forgotten). Remember to ask about potential GI side effects whenever any new medication is prescribed. As a caregiver, you may find it helpful to have stool softeners, laxatives, or even enemas on hand in case you may need to administer a remedy to a loved one (rather than having to run out to a pharmacy in the middle of the night). To avoid over- or underutilization, we recommend that a caregiver dispense these rather than relying on a patient with dementia to correctly self-administer. We often share with our patients and families the helpful adage: "If you don't move, your bowels won't move." Prevention and treatment of bowel irregularity usually work quite well. Avoidance does not.

Common sense rule: Patients with dementia can overdo medications due to forgetfulness, dependence, and/or other factors.

Illicit Drugs

We do not commonly encounter illegal substance abuse in our (mostly elderly) patients with dementia, however such drugs can cause or contribute to significant cognitive, behavioral, and other neuropsychiatric problems. In such cases, we recommend working with a specialist, an addiction specialist, if warranted. The same general principles apply as do for alcohol or overutilization of prescription drugs: A patient with dementia may be extremely susceptible to adverse effects of any substance, a patient's physician needs to be made aware of use or abuse of any drug (particularly when cognitive, behavioral, and other neuropsychiatric symptoms are being evaluated), and abrupt withdrawal without medical care may be dangerous or even deadly. This topic may become increasingly important in future generations in which such legally prohibited products have been more commonly used.

Medications Adverse to Memory

Many drugs can also interfere with memory (and cognitive enhancers), often by reducing available acetylcholine (i.e., the opposite of what the cognitive enhancing cholinesterase inhibitors do—see Chap. 8). Anticholinergic medications include drugs used to treat bladder incontinence, insomnia, and gastric reflux. This is by no means an exhaustive list of anticholinergic medication, and many other types of drugs, including other sedatives (sleep medications) and some antidepressants (especially the so-called "tricyclic antidepressants," like amitriptyline and nortriptyline), can also interfere with memory. Check with a patient's doctor and, preferably, a prescribing physician or specialist. For patients with dementia, it is crucial to work with a specialist or other doctor to identify any drugs that may be worsening the condition and avoiding or minimizing their use whenever possible.

Diphenhydramine (Trade name: Benadryl), either alone or in combination with another ingredient, represents the most common over-the-counter drug contributing to memory problems in our patients. Combination medications containing diphenhydramine often carry a "PM" designation in the trade name, such as Tylenol PM (which is acetaminophen + diphenhydramine) or Motrin PM (ibuprofen + diphenhydramine) or Advil PM (also ibuprofen + diphenhydramine). Diphenhydramine can also cause or exacerbate constipation and urinary retention for some people.

Patients over 65 are exquisitely sensitive to these effects. We often see some improvement in memory after stopping a medication containing diphenhydramine in our elderly patients. Even though some of these drugs can be obtained without a prescription, they should be listed on a patient's medication list. Dementia specialists avoid use of these products in dementia, whenever possible, due to their risk of causing or exacerbating memory loss or delirium. Delirium is a medical term used to describe altered mental status, fluctuating cognition, and confusion.

If patients take any of these products for pain, we recommend that they continue to take the pain ingredient without the diphenydramine (e.g., taking acetaminophen or brand name Tylenol alone rather than Tylenol PM).

If a patient with dementia has troubling insomnia after discontinuation of diphenydramine, a mild prescription sleep aid in small doses may be a better option and can be titrated up to higher doses as necessary. Trazodone (Trade name: Desyrel) is a sedative that can be initiated at a small dose of 50 mg and increased in increments of 25 mg. Side effects tend to be mild but may include dizziness and dry mouth. Priapism (prolonged erection) is a rare complication and less likely to occur in elderly men than younger men. Mirtazapine (Trade name: Remeron) is an antidepressant that also acts as a sedative. It can be started and titrated in increments of 7.5 mg. Side effects include increased appetite and weight gain, which may be advantageous in some elderly patients and those with dementia, who experience anorexia. Effects of increased weight and appetite actually lessen at higher doses of mirtazapine. Both trazodone and mirtazapine are available in generic form. Many other options exist and we strongly recommend working with a geriatric psychiatrist or other specialist to find the best solution targeting problematic symptoms (such as insomnia) that will avoid creating or worsening other ones (such as memory loss).

Is a Drug Exacerbating Dementia Symptoms?

Families frequently ask us whether a loved one with dementia has become more sedated, agitated, dizzy, hallucinating, etc., due to medication. Timing probably represents the most critical factor here. If a symptom starts or worsens in the hours or days after starting a new medication (or increasing the dosage of a medication), this suggests a temporal association. Such temporal relationships may also apply for alcohol or medications used intermittently. For example, a patient may be sedated on certain days of the week and careful review of medications and caregiver observation demonstrates that such somnolence occurs only in the mornings after the patient has had a sleeping pill at night. Or, a person with dementia may be hallucinating only on nights after having a glass of wine with dinner. Check with a patient's physician as to whether the two (the drug and the symptom) are related.

As noted in Chap. 8, even medications meant to "enhance" cognition can have side effects such as increased confusion. Associated symptoms (e.g., runny nose, sore throat, or cloudy urine), might also help in determining a cause, especially if it's been a while since any medication changes. For example, a patient might have an infection causing the symptom or symptoms.

Work with a patient's doctor to get to the root of the problem. As always, any necessary medication changes should be made cautiously and incrementally unless a significant medical rationale indicates otherwise. Any serious new medical condition deserves emergency evaluation.

Aluminum ≠ Alzheimer's

Finally, we would like to make a mention of aluminum. Although aluminum and Alzheimer's may sound like they should belong together (perhaps due to alliteration), scientific research has shown that aluminum does not cause AD [4], nor has it been associated with other types of dementia.

Summary

Alcohol in moderation is associated with reduced risk of dementia. Age and dementia increase susceptibility to drugs affecting brain function, including alcohol and medications. Opiates and sedatives represent two common classes of prescription medication on which patients may become dependent. Bowel products are also commonly overutilized. Many medications, but particularly anticholinergic agents like diphenhydramine, may impair memory. Temporal association may help identify whether and which drug/s may cause or contribute to a patient's symptoms.

Common Sense Rules

- Dementia may increase the effects of alcohol.
- Alcohol and drug withdrawal should be a gradual, supervised process.
- A patient's physician must be informed of alcohol intake.
- Regularly review the risks and benefits of alcohol and medications for a person with dementia.
- Patients with dementia can overdo alcohol or drugs due to forgetfulness, dependence, and/or other factors.
- Psychotherapy doesn't usually work for patients with significant dementia, but may help family caregivers.
- Maintain a daily routine for the person with dementia.
- Good sleep hygiene and pain management may alleviate some dementia symptoms.
- Even prescription drugs may be overutilized.
- Use sedating medications cautiously.
- A medication list helps avoid drug duplication.
- Memory functioning is critical for correct medication administration.
- Monitor medication administration and increase supervision as needed.

References

1. Neafsey EJ, Collins MA. Moderate alcohol consumption and cognitive risk. Neuropsychiatr Dis Treat. 2011;7(1):465–84.
2. Lopez OL, Becker JT, Sweet RA, et al. Psychiatric symptoms vary with the severity of dementia in probable Alzheimer's disease. J Neuropsychiatry Clin Neurosci. 2003;15(3):346–53.
3. Lyketsos CG, Lopez O, Jones B, Fitzpatrick AL, Breitner J, DeKosky S. Prevalence of neuropsychiatric symptoms in dementia and mild cognitive impairment: results from the cardiovascular health study. JAMA. 2002;288(12):1475–83.
4. Munoz DG, Feldman H. Causes of Alzheimer's disease. CMAJ. 2000;162(1):65–72. Review.

Part III
Mood and Behavior

Chapter 11
Mood Issues in Dementia

Psychiatric and behavioral changes go hand in hand with dementia. Psychiatric issues include problems with mood, anxiety, and psychosis. We defer the discussion on psychosis to the next chapter where we discuss the more common problematic behaviors we see in dementia.

Depression

Mood disturbance is common in Alzheimer's dementia. Depression occurs in approximately 40 % of Alzheimer's patients [1, 2]. The interaction between depression and dementia is complicated. We know that depression is a risk factor for Alzheimer's disease. We also know that a diagnosis of depression may precede the Alzheimer's diagnosis by several years. This is not surprising since the earliest signs of dementia may be social withdrawal and apathy—not memory.

Common sense rule: Social withdrawal or mood disturbance may be the first symptom of Alzheimer's Disease.

One question that comes up regularly in the office is whether the depression is causing the memory problems. Depression affects the attentional component of memory. The idea is as follows: if you are depressed, you cannot pay attention to the information well enough to learn it. If you do not learn the information efficiently, you cannot recall it. Therefore, memory looks impaired. In contrast, with Alzheimer's disease the memory mechanism itself is impaired. Attention is usually intact.

However, standard neuropsychological tests are sensitive enough to ascertain whether depression is contributing to memory disturbance. The concern is that when depression captures the focus of clinicians and family, an underlying dementia may go untreated.

A.M. Lipton and C.D. Marshall, *The Common Sense Guide to Dementia for Clinicians and Caregivers*, DOI 10.1007/978-1-4614-4163-2_11,
© Springer Science+Business Media, LLC 2013

Common sense rule: Significant forgetfulness is typically caused by a primary memory disorder.

Apathy/Emotional Blunting

Apathy is often confused with depression. When a loved one withdraws from socialization and former enjoyable activities, the assumption is that the person must be depressed. Typically the patient denies feeling sad and is not bothered by the level of withdrawal or inactivity. Apathy is a hard concept to wrap your head around. We often operationally define this as a someone who is content to sit in a chair all day. Emotional blunting refers to a lack of a person's affective response. (Remember mood is how one feels himself or herself. Affect is how he or she is perceived by others.) Someone with emotional blunting may not smile or laugh at appropriate junctures or reciprocate an expression or gesture of love, such as a hug, kiss, or "I love you". Emotional blunting may be associated with apathy, depression, dementia, or a combination. It is one of the hallmarks of FTD. Apathy is quite common in Alzheimer's disease with estimates around 60–70 % [3, 4]. As noted above, it may be the first major symptom of Alzheimer's disease.

Anxiety

Although studies do not attempt to define types of anxiety, we commonly see anxiety either be situational or generalized. The exact numbers are hard to quantify as its prevalence has been studied in whole and during different stages of dementia. Situational anxiety may be seen in patients early in disease who have heightened awareness of their deficits. They may become anxious when they struggle with a task that once came relatively easy to them. Maybe they are slower or less accurate. You may see more anxiety as the complexity of the task increases, such as completing a tax return. In later stages we may see patients become anxious whenever they leave their home, such as to go to a doctor's visit.

We also see more generalized symptoms. Patients typically describe this is as a general feeling of unease. They may not be able to identify anything in particular that makes them feel anxious. Or they may ruminate on anxiety-laden topics such as their various physical problems or their fear of running out of money. It is not uncommon to have a more advanced patient repeatedly ask others what they should be doing.

Irritability/Disinhibition

Irritability is regularly seen in Alzheimer's disease with estimates traditionally between 41 and 42 % [3, 4], as well as many other types of dementia. Families often describe the patient as being snappy, on edge, or having a short fuse. The irritability can be triggered by a frustrating event or may be fairly generalized. Hateful words may be uttered. Some may even start cursing or making derogatory comments about another's race, gender, or religion. The latter can be quite disturbing to families, particularly when viewed as out of character for their loved one.

Treatment

Depression may be treated with medications generally classified as antidepressants. Anxiety and/or irritability may also respond to nonstimulating antidepressants. When possible we avoid prescribing sedatives for anxiety in geriatric patients due to the increased risk for somnolence, confusion, and falls with these drugs.

The treatment of apathy is more challenging as response to medication is not robust. If medication is indicated, physicians tend to use categories of medication that increase availability of norepinephrine and dopamine in the brain. Simply put, these neurotransmitters are your "get up and go" chemicals. These medications include a subcategory of the antidepressant family as well as stimulants. Stimulants have a higher side effect profile, so they are used judiciously. In addition to known cardiac and appetite suppression effects, we must consider risk of psychosis and agitation in patients with underlying dementia.

We strongly recommend increased activity for the psychiatric symptoms of dementia. No one's apathy or depression improves with spending time alone and idle. The combination of meaningful activity and being around others lifts spirits.

Anxiety likewise thrives with inactivity. We caution our inactive anxious patients, "you have way too much time to spend in your own head." The brain uses all that free time to think, worry, and obsess.

Not having any luck getting your loved one involved in activity? Consider bringing in a companion to keep your loved one active. Often companions have a much easier time getting patients with dementia out and about than friends and family. Patients may display oppositional behavior towards relatives, but put on company manners for a professional caregiver. The structured activities and camaraderie afforded by adult day programs may work wonders for a patient, particularly one who is used to a daily job routine.

Common sense rule: Find ways to keep patients with dementia active.

Summary

Mood symptoms are common in dementia, but differ among individuals. These may include apathy, agitation, depression, and irritability. Treatment may include medications and nonpharmacologic approaches, such as social and other activity.

Common Sense Rules

- Social withdrawal or mood disturbance may be the first symptom of Alzheimer's disease.
- Significant forgetfulness is typically caused by a primary memory disorder.
- Find ways to keep patients with dementia active.

References

1. Wragg RE, Jeste DV. Overview of depression and psychosis in Alzheimer's disease. Am J Psychiatry. 1989;146:577–87.
2. Teng E, Ringman JM, Ross LK, et al; for the Alzheimer's Disease Research Centers of Californmia-Depression in Alzheimer's Diseases Investigators. Diagnosing depression in Alzheimer disease with the national institute of mental health provisional criteria. Am J Geriatr Psychiatry 2008;16(6):469–77
3. Lopez OL, Becker JT, Sweet RA, et al. Psychiatric symptoms vary with the severity of dementia in probable Alzheimer's disease. J Neuropsychiatry Clin Neurosci. 2003;15(3):346–53.
4. Mega MS, Cummings JL, Fiorello T, Gornbein J. The spectrum of behavioral changes in Alzheimer's disease. Neurology. 1996;46:130–5.

Chapter 12
Psychosis

Psychosis (Hallucinations and Delusions)

Psychosis refers to an affective condition in which a patient has lost touch with reality and has hallucinations, delusions, or both. The presence of psychosis in the initial months or year of a dementia suggests a non-Alzheimer's dementia or aggravating factor (such as medication) in the context of Alzheimer's disease.

Hallucinations

A hallucination is an abnormal sensory perception of a stimulus that isn't really there. The most common types of hallucinations in dementia are visual (seeing things), auditory (hearing something), or tactile (sensation of feeling something). In dementia, visual hallucinations are the most common, but auditory hallucinations may also occur. Tactile hallucinations suggest a different diagnosis than dementia. Hallucinations are a diagnostic criterion in Dementia with Lewy bodies and occur in approximately 10 % of patients with Alzheimer's dementia [1].

Delusions

A delusion is a fixed false belief that is resistant to reason or confrontation with facts. The take-home points from this formal definition are the words "fixed" and "false." Delusions may involve paranoia (in which a patient mistakenly believes that others are trying to inflict harm in some way). Delusions are estimated to occur in approximately 22 % of Alzheimer's dementia patients [1, 2].

A.M. Lipton and C.D. Marshall, *The Common Sense Guide to Dementia for Clinicians and Caregivers*, DOI 10.1007/978-1-4614-4163-2_12,
© Springer Science+Business Media, LLC 2013

Delusions of Theft

One of the most common examples that we encounter in our clinical practice is a dementia patient who experiences a delusion of theft. The patient mistakenly thinks that someone is entering the patient's residence and taking things or moving them around. Often what is actually occurring is that the patient with dementia is losing or hiding belongings from himself or herself.

When Mom asserts that there is someone coming into the home, the family often assumes that Mom is hallucinating. On further questioning, we often determine that Mom just thinks that there is someone in the house and is therefore having a delusion rather than a hallucination. She may cite evidence of the intruder, naming missing items or items being relocated within the home.

Let us walk through another common example. Dad has Alzheimer's disease, and one of his sons takes over managing Dad's financial affairs. The son oversees bank statements, pays bills, manages Dad's investments, etc. Dad becomes convinced that the son is stealing from him. The son provides Dad full access to the accounts to show him everything is being handled appropriately. Dad is unmoved by the information. Other family members go over bank statements with Dad to reassure him that all of his finances are in order. Dad continues to assert that son is stealing despite this evidence to the contrary.

Many families understandably struggle in these situations. Even when children are educated and insightful about the situation, it hurts to have your father accuse you of stealing. It may cause a rift in the parent–child relationship which is even more wounding. So what do you do? First realize the idea that son is stealing is fixed and false. Therefore, you can stop arguing with Dad. Deep down we often feel that we can convince Dad that he is wrong. And we can not. You can present document after document to prove your case. You can plead, argue, and threaten if you want. However, it typically does not bring resolution. As one of the children, when Dad tries to engage you in conversation about the stealing, provide one reassuring statement and change the subject. If you cannot change the course of the conversation, end the phone conversation or walk away. Of course you can consider other reasonable options, such as paying an accountant to manage Dad's affairs, as long as you realize the accusations may transfer to the new person.

But, if your loved one is experiencing psychosis, don't despair. As the above example shows, certain methods may be employed successfully. We offer a number of tips in the following sections to help you steer clear of what doesn't work and identify what will.

Addressing Psychosis

Here are a few techniques to keep in mind (and at hand) that you can draw on in a pinch.

First, provide comfort and reassurance. If your husband has a delusion that strangers are in the bedroom, remind him that you're with him and he's safe. You might turn on lights if it is dark or look around a room (including opening closet doors) with him so that he can see that any supposed intruders are no longer there ("Oh, look they're gone!") and you might make a show of checking any external door locks.

In addition to specific hallucinations and delusions, patients with dementia may have generalized paranoia. Alzheimer's patients may hide their valuables for fear they will be stolen. The memory deficits of this disease then impair the patient from remembering they hid the valuable. So this reinforces the paranoia as the object is actually missing. Families often file complaints with their loved one's living facility about missing items only to later discover them in a hiding place in their loved one's apartment. So, when Mom states her pearl earrings have been stolen, take a logical approach. Ideally you have an inventory of the belongings she took with her when she moved. First, verify if the earrings are listed on the inventory. The inventory alone saves a round of questioning about the missing item. Patients may get irritable if they feel family doubts them or questions their recall. If the earrings are on the inventory, carefully look through the entire apartment, not just where Mom keeps her jewelry. You might do so discreetly or together with Mom. If you have tried all of these measures and the earring still cannot be found, notify the administration.

Common sense rule: Support and reassure a patient with psychosis.

Think of hallucinations and delusions in the context of the brain sending aberrant signals. Unlike how hallucinations are portrayed in the movies, there is no halo around or hazy effect to the image. The brain signals that there is someone sitting across from Dad just as if there is one. That is why you cannot correct the misperception with words and it works best to avoid explanations, especially lengthy ones.

Instead of providing your thoughts on the matter ("Mom, I think you misplaced your earrings. I do not feel the staff is stealing.") opt for a strong declarative statement in attempts to end the discussion. You could try, "Mom, don't worry. I'm going to handle this." You don't have to provide specifics, such as that you're going to talk with the administrator, even if you are. Stay general but assertive. We recommend not engaging in lengthy conversations about the alleged theft. Paranoia is often driven by fear. We want Mom to feel reassured and know that you are looking out for her.

Don't correct, contradict, or otherwise confront or argue with a person who is having a hallucination or delusion. As a matter of fact, this is almost always a sound rule to follow for patients with dementia. All of these may just upset your loved one (and you will probably find it distressing as well).

Common sense rule: Avoid explanations or confrontation.

If you are going to address the psychosis head on, try a more medical interpretation to allay a patient's anxiety. You might gently remind Mom: "Remember, Dr. Smith said your mind may send some mixed-up signals sometimes." Then find an activity to engage the mind, preferably in another room. Distraction works well for psychosis and other behavioral problems. You can change the topic of conversation, activity, or even the venue. A snack may be just the thing. Changing the environment may help the brain let go of the image. You might take a patient to another room or even out of the house. This often works well for patients who are convinced that they aren't at home when in fact they are. After taking Mom to another room or place, you can bring her back and show her a couple of her favorite things (such as beloved photo, painting, or armchair), reassuring her that she is indeed home.

Common sense rule: Distraction works wonders.

Humor helps defuse potentially explosive situations. When you sense the conversation turning toward the delusional idea, insert a funny story about one of the grandkids. You might memorize some jokes, have a joke book handy in the house, or carry one with you. Laughter really is the best medicine.

Common sense rule: Humor defuses tension.

When Medication is Needed for Psychosis

Unfortunately, sometimes behavioral interventions are not enough for patients with psychosis. In these cases, the paranoia interferes with quality of life such that further action is needed. Maybe there is police involvement due to repeated calls from a patient reporting theft. Or maybe the paranoia leads to agitation that compromises the patient's ability to reside in his current level of care. Or maybe the patient is so burdened by her concerns that she will not leave her apartment for meals because would be leaving valuables unattended. There are no FDA-approved medications to treat dementia-related psychosis, but antipsychotic medications, which have FDA indications for other forms of psychosis, such as bipolar disorder and schizophrenia, may be used "off-label" if a patient is suffering. *Be advised that all antipsychotics carry a FDA boxed warning regarding their use in dementia.* The warning summarizes evidence that there is a 1.6- to 1.7-fold increased risk of death for dementia patients who take antipsychotic medication compared to those who do not. The studies that led to the FDA warning found the mechanism of death was mostly cardiac or pneumonia in origin. The antipsychotics also carry metabolic risks, such as increased blood sugar and cholesterol, as well as orthostatic risks, such as lowering blood pressure on standing. Sedation is also a risk for the majority of antipsychotics. We recommend a careful review, discussion, and consideration of the risks and benefits of such medication for any individual with dementia.

Summary

Patients with dementia may experience psychosis, which can include hallucinations or delusions. Hallucinations involve an abnormal sensory perception, whereas delusions portend fixed, false ideas. Minimizing any identifiable triggers may help prevent psychosis. Caregivers should offer comfort and safety for the person experiencing psychosis while sidestepping any arguments, conflict, or confrontation through the use of distraction and other behavioral and environmental measures. Antipsychotic medication may be prescribed for patients with dementia, but have known and serious risks which should be carefully considered.

Common Sense Rules

- Identify and avoid behavioral triggers.
- Avoid explanations or confrontation.
- Find the right balance of stimulation.
- Maintain a daily routine of structured activities.
- Support and reassure a patient with psychosis.
- Distraction works wonders.
- Humor defuses tension.

References

1. Mega MS, Cummings JL, Fiorello T, Gornbein J. The spectrum of behavioral changes in Alzheimer's disease. Neurology. 1996;46:130–5.
2. Bassiony MM, Steinberg MS, Warren A, Rosenblatt A, Baker AS, Lyketsos CG. Delusions and hallucinations in Alzheimer's disease: prevalence and clinical correlates. Int J Geriatr Psychiatry. 2000;15:99–107.

Chapter 13
Dealing with Problem Behaviors in Dementia

Many behavioral issues accompany dementia. These may be associated with psychosis and/or mood problems, such as depression, anxiety, apathy, and irritability—all of which have been defined in previous chapters. Some patients have minimal bothersome behaviors, and some will have many. In either case, it helps to have an understanding of these, as well as when, if, and HOW to intervene.

We find many families unsure as to whether problem behaviors (e.g., napping during the day) that they may observe in a loved one with dementia are related to disease or perhaps another reason, such as medication side effects. Sometimes multiple factors may be involved. We therefore itemize behavioral issues below which may be associated with dementia. We also include relevant medication issues and numerous techniques to tackle behavioral troubles. These may include adding, altering, or removing medications, but focus on nonpharmacologic measures that any caregiver may administer.

Behavioral Triggers

People with dementia may have troubles with mood or behavior without any apparent reason (other than the illness itself). However, sometimes, a "trigger" for problem behaviors can be identified. This might be an event or task, a noise or conversation, an object or other visual item, a medication, or even a person or time of day. Sometimes even items meant to be cheerful or merely decorative, such as holiday trimmings or mirrors, may disturb someone with dementia. Try to identify and avoid such triggers, wherever possible. This can obviously pose difficulties, especially if someone with dementia becomes aggravated with a caregiver or other close person who can't be replaced. In such cases, consider changing tone of voice, approach (a hug instead of an explanation) and/or enlisting the help of others.

A.M. Lipton and C.D. Marshall, *The Common Sense Guide to Dementia for Clinicians and Caregivers*, DOI 10.1007/978-1-4614-4163-2_13,
© Springer Science+Business Media, LLC 2013

An "overstimulating" environment might include a number of such behavioral triggers, such as crowds, noise, visual information, and clutter. It often helps to maintain a quiet, calm atmosphere—or have one in mind if it becomes necessary (say, prearranging to use a back room at a large party). Decluttering a home and cleaning out closets may be desirable (and perhaps best done when the person with behavioral issues is not present, so as to avoid the problem you are trying to prevent). Since people with dementia often remember the past better than the here and now, you may wish to pack away items before permanently removing them, as an old favorite may be missed and need to be returned to its usual place. Sometimes an unfamiliar setting can completely overwhelm a person with dementia, so keep these principles in mind for trips, hospitalizations, and the like. These precepts are particularly valuable in caring for patients with impulsive behaviors/disinhibition which may develop into irritability, agitation, or aggression. The level of stimulation that works best varies for each individual, by stage of dementia, and sometimes from day to day. Let your loved one be your guide.

Common sense rule: Minimize behavioral triggers.

Repetitive Behavior

A variety of excessively repetitive or *perseverative* behaviors may occur in dementia. These are often associated with anxiety and/or agitation. They may stem from forgetfulness (and falling back on old habits), personality changes, or both. *Compulsions* involve an overwhelming urge to have or do something a certain way. A compulsion may represent relatively innocuous behavior, such as setting the table in a fixed arrangement, or a more consequential one, such as gambling. *Punding* refers to collecting, tinkering, and sorting behaviors. Some other specific types of repetitive behaviors, such as pacing and scratching, are addressed later in this chapter. Asking the same question over and over again occurs commonly in Alzheimer's disease and other dementias. An individual with poor short-term memory displays problems learning and remembering new information.

Let us be frank here. Repetitive questioning is very annoying and leads to caregiver frustration and anger. Yet, we would caution against telling your loved one that you have already answered that question five times over. When you give that feedback, your loved one, who truly does not remember asking the first four times, receives a verbal critique as well as a reminder that his or her memory is poor. Sometimes the memory of a negative emotion is retained much longer than the original item to be remembered. Criticism can also lead to agitation. Avoid negative remarks and employ the strategies mentioned below (or exercise your ingenuity and implement one of your own).

Common sense rule: Refrain from reprimands.

It's OK to answer the question, even more than once, but not to the point that it becomes annoying (or worse) to you. This threshold will be different for everyone, but try to find a different tactic before you reach your boiling point. Instead of giving another verbal response that will be forgotten, try writing down the answer. It is common for patients with dementia to repeatedly ask about the day, date, or daily activities. Try to prevent this by keeping an easily visible wall calendar (and/or whiteboard/dry-erase board) in the house so you can record activities and appointments. When asked which doctor you're seeing today for the third time, refer your loved one to the calendar. You do not have to answer the question over and over, nor should you. Simple tactics can address all types of repetitive behaviors. Take a break. Change the subject. Try distraction. Get your loved one involved in a chore or grab the phone and help him call a friend.

Common sense rule: You do not have to answer the same question over and over.

Agitation/Irritability/Disinhibition

When your loved one starts to escalate, back off. Often family members inadvertently get themselves into a precarious situation by arguing with a loved one. Unfortunately, although you will eventually calm down, your loved one with dementia may not. But, if he or she has a poor memory, you might try walking away for a few minutes and see if the reason for getting so upset is forgotten.

Employ the common sense rules of balancing stimulation and providing distraction. Have some calming activities close by. Break up the agitation by asking Mom to fold the laundry. Sometimes you don't even have to say anything. Just put the laundry basket in the room with Mom. Have favorite music ready to play.

Many times our loved ones give us clues as to what situations they can and cannot handle. Avoid situations that caused problems in the past, such as noisy restaurants. As a general rule, avoid overstimulation. Have family visit one or two at a time versus scheduling a family dinner, particularly if young children will be present. When agitation cannot be controlled with medication or environmental modification, it often becomes the driving force in moving someone with dementia to a memory care facility.

Aggression/Combativeness

Aggression may be verbal, physical, and/or sexual. Verbal aggression may include hateful words, name-calling, racial slurs, screaming, and/or cursing. Physical aggression may be directed at inanimate objects (e.g., breaking or throwing things) or towards people (e.g., hitting or biting). Sexual aggression may manifest as something like trying to grab a woman's bosom.

Try to identify and avoid any possible triggers of such behavior. For example, if sexual aggression is directed at a spouse in a sheer nightgown, switching to pajamas with more coverage may help. Combativeness may occur in response to being physically coerced or forced to do something, such as being led to the shower. In advanced dementia, your loved one may not comprehend what you or another caregiver wants them to do. Imagine how you would feel if someone tried to lead you by the arm and you didn't understand why. You would probably instinctively try to flee the person's grasp or fight back. Since the mental status of patients with dementia tends to decline as the day goes on, we recommend scheduling necessary activities in the morning as much as possible. This includes such things as showers and doctor's appointments. And, instead of taking Mom by the arm, you might try sitting down with her and then seeing if she gets up when you do and will follow you. If she needs more support or guidance, you might try holding hands with her after a moment of sitting down in a relaxed state and then rise together.

In memory care facilities, aggression may be triggered by paranoia. Maybe a peer wandered into Dad's room, and he fought them as he would an intruder breaking in his home. Following common sense rules to find and minimize any such behavioral trigger may help reduce such behavior.

Scratching, Picking, and Slapping

Scratching, picking, and slapping (or hitting oneself) may be self-comforting or self-stimulating behaviors for a patient with dementia, but can generate considerable anguish for family members and other caregivers. We have seen patients scratch and pick at their skin until it bleeds. And the process may be repeated over and over, including for any scabs that form. Consultation with a dermatologist and a trial of anti-itching pills and creams may be warranted, especially since patients exhibiting these behaviors may have advanced dementia and difficulty communicating symptoms. However, despite a common assumption that such patients are scratching to relieve an itching sensation, they often do not appear to be in any distress and will stop itching if distracted. Oral anti-itching medications also often have side effects of sedation and memory impairment. Nonetheless, a dermatologist can provide a significant degree of support and reassurance by ruling out any underlying skin condition and guiding good skin care, including treatment and prevention of further skin damage, infection, etc.

From a pharmacological standpoint, we can utilize medications for obsessive-compulsive behaviors, but these are also unlikely to be very effective. These behaviors are also not particularly responsive to caregivers reminding or reprimanding patient ("Don't do that"). The best treatments are the common sense ones, such as distraction. Here are some specific ways to address scratching, picking, and slapping:

- Keep nails clipped short.
- Give a patient something, such as flexible ball or a washcloth, to hold or squeeze in one or both hands (or give the patient something else to do with the hands).

- Long-sleeved clothing often works well, especially shirts with sleeves that are difficult to unbutton and/or roll up.
- Light cotton gloves may be worn.
- Keep skin moisturized with lotion to prevent easy skin tearing.

In severe cases, the affected area may be dressed with bandages that are hard to remove. The family of one of our patients successfully used an arm sleeve that was designed to protect burn victims' skin.

Sundowning/Confusion

"Sundowning" connotes the confusion and other symptoms often observed in dementia patients, particularly those with Alzheimer's disease, as the sun goes down. Increased disorientation, emotional lability, agitation, resistance to care, and combativeness may occur. Sundowning may begin earlier in the afternoon or later in the evening than the actual time of sunset, but it often starts around the same time each day for a given individual with dementia. Note this timing as it may direct when medication should be given. For patients who require medication to manage any of these symptoms, we try to dose it prior to the typical hour of "sundowning." Consider moving any or all of a patient's other drugs to this time or earlier, if possible, since a patient may refuse to take medication after "sundowning."

A sudden onset or worsening of confusion may indicate an infection. A urinary tract infection, in particular, is a common cause of an acute mental status change. This may need to be assessed in an emergency department or by a primary care physician, depending on the speed and severity of the change.

Pacing/Excessive Walking/Abnormal Motor Behavior

Some patients with dementia show a need to pace or walk. We suspect this release of energy is beneficial for the patient and generally encourage it with protected freedom (i.e., a supervised enclosed walking area or walking with a responsible adult). Alert a patient's physician about this behavior, as "akathisia" may be a side effect of certain medications, particularly some those to treat psychosis or nausea. Akathisia may be described as an internal restlessness and need to move. Patients with akathisia literally "can't sit still. Since it may be difficult to ascertain whether the pacing is consistent with a dementia behavior or a medication side effect, it is important for your physician to see and assess the movement. If it happens on-and-off, you might take a video, so that you have something to show the doctor (in case the motor problems don't occur at the time of a clinic visit).

Wandering

No drug will prevent patients with dementia from leaving home or wandering away in public, so alternative measures should be employed. Since safety is paramount, we recommend installing door alarms for all exterior doors. The alarm will alert others in the home if your loved one tries to exit. You can use bells on internal and external doorknobs as a cheaper, low-tech solution (if you are a light sleeper). You can also try disguising a door with a poster or something similar, so that it is not as obvious as an exit.

When door alarms are not sufficient, consider keyed locks on the interior of all doors that open to the outside of the home. The location of the key must be kept secret from your loved one with dementia who wanders. Fortunately, most patients will try a locked door and move on when it does not open. However, you must weigh the risk of being locked in your home in case of fire or other emergency in which you would need to exit the home without delay.

Repeated wandering represents a risk to basic safety and a need for placement in a secure (locked) memory care facility. Even the most diligent caregiver cannot supervise a loved one 24 h a day.

Several services can help you locate a person with dementia missing outside the home. You must enroll for each service and pay the appropriate monthly fee. The MedicAlert® + Alzheimer's Association Safe Return℠ program pairs an identification pendant with a 24 h emergency response service. If a loved one goes missing, family reports it to the emergency response number. The program then notifies local law enforcement. For a concerned citizen or first responder who finds your loved one, the identification necklace or bracelet provides the emergency contact number and the information that your loved one has memory.

In addition, companies have employed advanced technology to create locator services for patients with dementia. The Alzheimer's Association Comfort Zone™ is a web based location management service that utilizes global positioning system (GPS) technology. The locator device resembles a pager or cell phone, and your loved one must carry the device with him/her (presumably via purse or pocket or mounted in a car). Therefore, this device would be most useful in earlier stages of dementia. Various options are available, including tracking and alerts when your loved one travels outside a preset zone.

EmFinders® produces the EmSeeQ® product, a watch-like device utilizing cellular technology to locate a missing patient with dementia. When a loved one goes missing, the registered caregiver notifies 911 and the EmFinders Operations Center. The Operations Center activates the device which literally calls 911 with a preset message and its location. It may be purchased with a secure band which requires a two-hands approach to remove it, so that a patient cannot remove it without assistance.

Finally, the Silver Alert system has been adopted by many states to aid in the return of missing elderly with dementia, particularly those traveling by car. Modeled after the AMBER Alert system for child abduction, this service involves broadcasting pertinent information about the missing person, such as description of car, city of origin, and license plate number via radio, television, and electronic roadway signs. When a car is involved, it is not unusual for a person to be found a hundred or more miles away. And, although it should go without saying, once your loved one heads off to the dentist and ends up in another city, it is time to take away the car.

Common sense rule: Take safety precautions to prevent wandering.

Problems in Unfamiliar Surroundings

A patient with dementia may become disoriented and agitated, as well as less functional in an unfamiliar environment, such as in a hospital or on a trip. This may occur even in a place, such as a relative's home, that he or she has stayed at before and may be worse at night (see section on "Sundowning" above). Essentially, the person cannot navigate removed from the familiar anchor of home. He or she may seem more irritable or confused, perhaps found sitting in the kitchen in the wee hours of the morning after not being able to find a bathroom. Tasks easily performed previously, such as dressing, bathing, and shaving, may become difficult outside the usual routine. A situation that causes distress in person with dementia or caregiver signals that the patient should stop traveling (e.g., wandering out of a hotel room in a state of undress). Out-of-town family should visit the patient rather than vice versa. Caregivers may continue to travel (and it may be an important and healthy break for them—and their loved ones—for them to do so) so long as arrangements can be made for other relatives or professional caregivers to take care of the patient, either in the home or via respite care at a care facility. (see Chap. 15: Selecting Level of Care for further information on respite care.) Veterans may be eligible for at least a couple of weeks of respite care annually through the Veterans Administration program.

Common sense rule: Patients with dementia may decompensate in unfamiliar environments.

Disruption of Sleep–Wake Cycle

As dementia progresses, it may produce a disturbance in a patient's sleep–wake cycle, with increased napping during the day and less sleep at night. Although often attributed to medication, drugs for dementia do not typically cause somnolence. However, some medications may, especially those used to treat insomnia or other behavioral problems. These include sedatives and sedating antipsychotics.

Daytime activity is the best way to combat daytime sedation. Many people nod off because they sit around all day. Likewise, the best way to sleep well at night is to stay active during the day and avoid excessive napping. Rather than allowing a loved one doze off at any time, we recommend scheduling short (30–60 min) naps just like other daily activities, perhaps at a natural siesta time after lunch. Dementia specialists are cautious about using traditional sleep medication in dementia, due to increased risk of falls, confusion, and memory impairment.

Good sleep hygiene is key. Patients (and caregivers!) should stick to regular bedtimes, nap times, and morning reveille. Gradually reduce activity and stimuli towards nightfall, including light and noise. Set the stage for slumber by helping your loved one dress for bed. Provide a typical bedtime snack of milk and cookies. Turn down lights and bed covers. Speak in a soft voice (or even tell a bedtime story), play restful music or maintain complete quiet, depending on what works best to induce somnolence. A hand massage with scented lotion can also be soothing and sleep-inducing.

Common sense rule: Schedule daily activities and routine times for sleep.

Poor Appetite/Sweet Tooth

Loss of appetite is a tough issue to address because it can be caused by dementia itself as well as by one category of medication used to treat the disease. Patients with dementia may have difficulty shopping, preparing meals, or remembering to eat, so caregivers should monitor and address these issues first.

All cholinesterase inhibitors (including donepezil, galantamine, and rivastigmine) carry a risk of anorexia. Therefore, inform the doctor of any decreased appetite or weight loss, especially prior to starting any new drugs. Discuss the risks and benefits of trying the medication with the physician. If symptoms began after the medication was started, the medication may be stopped to see if appetite improves. If the loss of appetite does not improve off medication, it may be prudent to resume the medication. Patient and family wishes weigh prominently here.

Some evidence suggests that appetite stimulants help with weight gain, but may add little to survival or functioning level. We don't recommend appetite stimulants or feeding tubes in patients with advanced dementia (see Chap. 16: Looking Ahead for further details).

Another common finding in dementia is a preference for sweets. A patient may refuse a well-balanced meal, but consume ice cream as if it is going out of style. If a patient younger than 65 years of age with dementia exhibits excessive consumption of food, especially sweets, as well as weight gain, this raises concern for a possible Frontotemporal dementia. For patients who overeat, it is best to mete out healthy portions. For example, plate the food in the kitchen rather than serving large dishes "family style" at the table. To address excessive snacking, limit free access to food and use small snack bags. High sugar consumption may cause significant weight gain, cavities, and even diabetes, so consider sugar-free substitutions for items like gum, candy, mints, and beverages.

In most other types of dementia, including Alzheimer's disease, patients are more likely to experience weight loss even with an increased preference for sweets. Sometimes small snacks or meals appear less overwhelming and are more readily consumed. You may have to be creative and add sugar to green beans to get a loved one with dementia to eat his or her vegetables. And, although we have to consider risks of diabetes and other health issues, for folks with advanced dementia, quality of life wins out. So—let them eat ice cream!

Common sense rule: Provide healthy meals.

Crying/Mood Swings

Emotional lability refers to rapid mood swings and may occur in dementia, especially non-Alzheimer's types. Regular crying spells occur in a subset of patients with dementia and other neurological illnesses, including strokes and traumatic brain injury. Such symptoms are understandably very disturbing for families. The crying may not be related to depression or triggered by anything in particular. Some patients have similar spells of laughing. Even though laughter may be easier to take than tears, it can still be disconcerting, especially when it occurs at inappropriate times (or much of the time), and impedes normal activity and conversation. Patients with severe emotional lability, who burst into tears and/or laughter at "the drop of a hat," may have a clinical syndrome known as Pseudobulbar affect. Activities, distraction, and certain medications, including antidepressants, may be extremely helpful in ameliorating emotional lability.

Noncompliance with Medication

Patients with dementia may forget to take their medication, but they may also refuse medication administered by family or other caregivers. They may verbally refuse, respond with pursed lips, or spit out the pills. There is no easy answer for this. Caregivers can walk away and try again later. As we discussed above, the mind does best in the morning. So, we can try to dose as medications early in the day. We can also trim down the medication list to a minimum. Ask your loved one's doctor (s) if any medications can be stopped or else given earlier in the day. Administer the most important drugs first. Many pills can be crushed (or capsules emptied) and placed in small amounts of food (such as a snack-size yogurt or pudding cup) as long as the drugs are not long-acting in nature. Check with a patient's physician and pharmacist about such options.

Common sense rule: Medications work best when taken regularly.

Refusal to Bathe/Change Clothes

Generally as dementia progresses, patients show less interest in hygiene. (The exception is patients with Frontotemporal dementia, who may demonstrate poor hygiene very early in the clinical course of their disease, even in the first few months or year.) Some patients with dementia will agree to sponge bathe, but will not get in the tub or shower. Hygiene is important in preventing infection. And, since urinary tract infections can play havoc on the brain and behavior, we prioritize basic hygiene, but compromise on frequency. Sometimes, a caregiver of patients with dementia may be advised to "pick your battles." We prefer to avoid conflict, whenever possible, and our recommendation is that you "pick your baths."

Often, we can utilize longstanding ideas that one has to bathe and dress up for an event or appointment or change clothes because they're "dirty." Try to present the bath or changing clothes in a way in which the patient does not feel forced or coerced. We essentially want the patient to think that it is his or her idea. You might act like you could care less, but pick phrasing that you know will motivate your loved one. Don't overwhelm with choices. Pick colorful clothes and favorite outfits that are easy to wear and present one (or a choice between just two shirts or tops) to the patient. Sometimes patients with dementia are more agreeable to bathing or dressing with a companion or aide than a family member. (This may be due to a particular rapport between individuals, ingrained social morays of not wanting to disrobe in front of a relative, patients putting on their "company manners," or a patient's wish to comply respectfully with medical or nursing professionals.)

Common sense rule: Pick your baths.

Pharmacologic Treatment

No medications are currently approved by the Food and Drug Administration (FDA) for the treatment of agitation or behavioral problems in dementia. However, physicians can intervene with medications using a systematic and logical approach. The most common categories of drugs used are as follows:

1. Antidepressants. Nonstimulating antidepressants may be beneficial and preferable to use ahead of other drugs with greater side effects.
2. Sedatives. These medications have significant side effects (including the sedation itself), but may be utilized to decrease agitation.
3. Antipsychotics. In the last chapter, we discussed the use of antipsychotic medication in greater detail. *All antipsychotics carry a FDA warning regarding their use in dementia.*

With all medication choices, physicians, patients, and families must weigh the benefit-to-risk ratio and quality of life considerations. For patients with severe agitation, we may utilize the sedating properties of medication to calm mind and body.

During discussion of such medication, families often express concern about "drugging Mom" or "turning Mom into a zombie." None of us want to see Mom overly sedated, but we also don't wish to see her in a state of distress if her brain gives us clear signals that it is overexcited and needs to calm down. In severe agitation, there is a long way to go from a state of excessive stimulation to somnolence. Dosage should "start low and go slow" with adjustments made along the way, including reducing or stopping medication for too much sedation.

Behavioral Interventions

The first intervention is prevention. Agitation and behavioral issues are intrinsic to this disease. Therefore, it is not realistic to expect that we can always prevent behavioral symptoms. *Second, identify early signs and intervene before your loved one escalates into a state of more significant agitation. Act when you see the thunderclouds roll in. Don't wait for lightning to strike.* The crafty caregiver uses knowledge, flexibility, and creativity to create a calm and appropriate response that serves to distract and redirect a loved one.

Common sense rule: The first intervention is prevention.

Take care of yourself. In this illness, the struggling brain gloms onto the person whose brain is functioning better. If you start to decline, so will your loved one. Maintain a regular routine. Avoid or reduce behavioral triggers and overstimulation. Keep outings short. Minimize evening commitments. Do not correct or argue with your loved one. Bring in help so that you don't become overly frustrated.

Common sense rule: Your loved one will only do as well as you are doing.

Learn about this disease. Then you can learn how to respond to your loved one with this disease. You are clearly committed to that path if you are reading this book. The next step, if you have not already done so, is to attend a caregiver class or caregiver series through the Alzheimer's Association. You can find your local chapter by going to the national website (www.alz.org) and entering your zip code when prompted. Your local chapter website will list upcoming classes and support groups. Both the national and local chapter Websites provide educational materials. Don't use a computer? Call the Alzheimer's Association 24 h helpline at 1888-272-3900.

Common sense rule: Educate yourself.

Probably the most useful behavioral intervention a caregiver can learn is the ability to distract from an unwanted emotional state or behavior and redirect toward a more desirable one. We never want to be patronizing to our elders or treat them like children. However, some principles that apply to the developing brain can also apply to the deteriorating brain. Our early school programs provide a structured day with good reason. Developing minds thrive on routine. Most parents go to great lengths to make sure their little ones do not get too tired or too hungry. Because, if they let their young one skip a nap or stay up late, they usually paid a high price for it. Furthermore, when is the last time you saw a Dad providing an extensive explanation to his toddler? Or a Mom arguing a point with her preschool age daughter? Choose your battles. Better yet, avoid them altogether. When a child asserts the sky is green, a parent might instinctively nod along versus arguing or repeatedly correcting.

Common sense rule: Distraction works wonders.

Rigidity is the enemy of caregiving success. So, if you have a hard time being flexible, this is going to be a hard road for you. Modify your strategy and expectations to the level your loved one is functioning at currently. We realize this is hard. We often observe what might be best characterized as a grief response when we see spouses make this transition. But, by accepting the changes and making these adjustments, you will change your life for the better.

Common sense rule: Be flexible.

Use simple sentences. Don't offer too many choices. Instead of asking your husband what he wants to wear, ask if he wants to wear the blue shirt or the green shirt. Is Dad not making much sense after 4 p.m.? Instead of repeatedly trying to clarify what he is saying, just nod along or periodically interject affirming words (such as "sure," "of course," etc.) to let him know that you're listening. If Mom starts ruminating about how her kids are stealing her savings, change the subject. Is Dad angrily demanding to speak with the bank manager about his accounts when he just did so yesterday? Try responding with vague, affirmative statements such as:

> "I've got to get on that. Thanks for reminding me."
> "I don't want you to worry, Dad. I'll take care of it."
> "Yes, I need to check on that. I'll let you know as soon as I hear something."

Can't get Dad off the subject? Try redirecting him to another activity. ("Sure we can go to the bank later, but I need to take out the trash and run to the store. Can you help?") Find what works for your loved one.

Common sense rule: Be simple and direct. And then, redirect!

Have activities on hand, emphasizing the favorite and familiar. For patients with moderate-to-advanced dementia, these might include:

- Sorting by color (helpful hint: candies are well received).
- Redistributing objects (placing coins or marbles into a jar).
- Simple chores (setting table, dusting, folding laundry).
  - Music ready to play with a touch of a button.
  - Movies or TV shows ready to play with touch of a button.

- Singing.
- Provide a baby doll to hold and care for (especially for patients who talk about or look for a "baby" or "babies," perhaps as part of confusion, delusions, or remembering the past).
- Hold tactile soothing objects (stuffed animals, soft blanket).
- Planting (indoors or out).
- Bake cookies with you operating the stove and mixer, allow loved one to pour ingredients and stir.
- Sit on the porch and watch the birds or have a glass of lemonade.
- Playing ball (tossing back and forth, toss ball into homemade hoop).
- Bring out old photos or even pull a picture off the wall to reminisce about family members or past times.
- Simple hobbies (coloring, painting, jigsaw puzzle—try to keep content age-appropriate but at a level commensurate with the patient's abilities. (In other words, it is OK to shop in the children's section, but perhaps purchase the puzzle with a picture of a landscape instead of a cartoon character.)

Remember that accuracy is not important and that a person with dementia may enjoy or even find comfort in repeating the same task. Consider leaving some items out that may attract your loved one to engage in activity independently in lieu of suggesting an activity. These might include a basket of laundry, a dust cloth on the table, or a stack of plates and napkins on the kitchen counter so that the patient may fold clothes, dust, or set the table. (And, you can take a load of spare clothes or towels to another room, mix them up, and return to your loved one to fold again and again.)

Common sense rule: Be creative.

Always consider memory day programs, which are described in more detail in Chap. 15: Selecting Level of Care. These offer activities throughout the day in a group setting. Individuals tend to join in because everyone else is participating. And caregivers get a break, too!

At the end of the day, behavioral issues can easily overwhelm a caregiver. Since the structured environment of memory care facilities can help, always keep this option open (including for temporary respite). Unfortunately, some families feel that having to move a loved one with dementia equates with failure or giving up, and we empathize with such sentiments. However, we have often observed, that when the time comes for such a move, waiting may impose significant strain on both patient and family, whereas a transition to memory care frequently represents a positive step toward greater stability and quality of life for all.

Summary

Behavioral problems regularly occur in dementia and can be addressed by a number of nonpharmacological means, as well as by medications in some cases. A caregiver can benefit from knowledge about dementia and a positive, flexible attitude. Creative solutions optimize health, safety, and activity level for the patient with dementia. Both a patient and caregiver can gain from implementation of behavioral and environmental measures.

Common Sense Rules

- Minimize behavioral triggers.
- Refrain from reprimands.
- You do not have to answer the same question over and over.
- Take safety precautions to prevent wandering.
- Patients with dementia may decompensate in unfamiliar environments.
- Schedule daily activities and routine times for sleep.
- Provide healthy meals.
- Medications work best when taken regularly.
- Pick your baths. The first intervention is prevention.
- Your loved one will only do as well as you are doing.
- Distraction works wonders.
- Educate yourself.
- Be flexible.
- Be simple and direct. And then, redirect!
- Be creative.

Part IV
Additional Considerations
in Dementia Care

Chapter 14
Legal and Financial Matters

"It is much better to prepare your wills, than to have a battle of them."

—Anne M. Lipton, M.D., Ph.D.

Introduction

We have often seen patients and families suffer significant emotional, medical, and financial consequences from failing to put legal powers in place. We therefore provide some basic information and definitions to help you in seeking and making the most of legal consultation.

Consulting an Attorney

We must start this chapter with a disclaimer: We are not attorneys. Since families regularly ask us about medicolegal issues, we hope to provide some perspective and clarity from our experience as dementia specialists, but it is imperative that you consult an attorney for legal advice. We realize the reassurance of working with a known and trusted personal/family attorney may outweigh the advantages afforded by a legal specialist. However, for our patients with dementia, we generally recommend consulting an elder law attorney who specializes in the legal needs of the aging population. How can you find such an attorney? Your personal attorney can recommend an elder law colleague. Your local Alzheimer's Association chapter or similar organization may have a list of local elder law attorneys. Another source would be the National Academy of Elder Law Attorneys (www.naela.org) which has an online search option. In addition, the Alzheimer's Association publishes a helpful brochure titled "Legal Plans" that can be accessed online (www.alz.org/national/documents/brochure_legalplans.pdf) [1].

A.M. Lipton and C.D. Marshall, *The Common Sense Guide to Dementia for Clinicians and Caregivers*, DOI 10.1007/978-1-4614-4163-2_14,
© Springer Science+Business Media, LLC 2013

Common sense rules:

- Consult an attorney for legal advice.
- Consider an attorney's specialty and experience regarding legal issues in dementia.

Definitions

Let's start by going over a few terms and what they mean. We have tried our best to convey the practical meaning and relevance of often confusing terminology in order to help caregivers of individuals with dementia. We have therefore primarily defined our terms operationally as they relate to patients, families, clinicians, and caregivers. These by no means substitute for complete legal definitions, particularly regarding capacity and competency. Such terms and their meanings may also vary by state or other jurisdiction or other context.

Capacity

Capacity is the ability to understand information relevant to a decision and to appreciate the reasonably foreseeable consequences of a decision or lack of decision [2]. Physicians may be asked (by attorneys, families, courts, and the like) to assess a person's capacity to comprehend and carry out certain functions, such as financial management or medical consent. Since capacity is specific to an activity, a person may have capacity to do one thing (consent to surgery) but not another (change a will). And, just because a person has dementia does not automatically mean he or she lacks capacity.

Common sense rule: Someone with dementia is not automatically incapacitated.

Competency

Competency is a legal designation—not a medical one. A person is presumed competent unless deemed otherwise by the court. Therefore, physicians cannot pronounce someone incompetent. Only a judge can make that declaration. We will explain this more fully later in the chapter.

Power of Attorney

In general, a POA document allows a person to appoint another person to act on his or her behalf. Since it can be constructed in a variety of ways, and because a POA addresses significant issues (such as financial, legal, and/or medical), this should be done so with care and legal guidance. We will discuss Medical POA in greater detail later in this chapter.

Advanced Health Care Directive (Living Will)

An advanced health care directive states what type of medical care an individual does and doesn't want if unable to voice his or her wishes. This typically includes preferences regarding life support and limits of medical care.

Guardianship and Conservatorship

If a court deems a person incapacitated, and the incapacitated person has no legal powers in place, the court may appoint a guardian or conservator. The term and the process vary from state to state, so it is important to work with an attorney who practices in the state where the alleged incapacitated person resides. For simplicity, we use the term guardian.

Constructing Your Legal Documents

The take-home message of this chapter is that each of us, not just those with dementia, benefits from having legal powers in place prior to any potentially incapacitating illness. We strongly recommend that you prepare your legal documents when you are well in mind and body—and without delay! Such documents should include an advanced health care directive (living will), POA including medical POA, and wills.

It serves everyone better to have Powers of Attorney and wills in place when they are needed than the unfortunate familial conflict and/or legal battles that may otherwise ensue. Avoid compounding the grief inherent to illness and death with further emotional and legal costs. We have seen families torn asunder (and spend untold sums) by divisiveness stemming from a patient's unknown and/or undocumented wishes for end-of-life care. In law, as in medicine, as in life itself, prevention of a crisis situation is best. And, if you can't prevent it, at least prepare for it. Your family and medical team thank you in advance.

Common sense rules:

- Only you can designate your POA.
- Everyone should get their legal affairs in order and make end-of-life wishes known.

But, in the real world, we often see patients who have no legal powers in place. Remember, someone with dementia is not necessarily incapacitated. A person who can understand and execute a decision can put powers in place. If the person has capacity to do so, we recommend the person meet with an elder law attorney to implement a POA and advanced health directives. And, although this is beyond the scope of this chapter, remember to review or create wills and/or trusts, as needed.

With regard to dementia, it is imperative to construct the power of attorney so that it is valid during periods of incapacity. If you are named as POA for someone no longer capable of making his or her own decisions, you may have to provide documentation to invoke this authority. Unfortunately, banks and other institutions vary in the documents required to prove a patient's incapacity and invoke a POA. Some require one doctor's note, while others require a letter from two separate physicians. Also, the wording that is acceptable to one institution may not be acceptable to another. Therefore, check on the documentation needed prior to any visit or phone call to a doctor's office, so that you can request it easily and exactly on the first go-around, saving everyone's time and effort.

As a caregiver for someone with dementia, we also recommend meeting with an attorney to create, review, and/or modify your own legal documents as needed. Remember what we said in Chap. 7 about caring for the caregiver first? It's bad enough if the patient with dementia doesn't have legal powers in place. What if something happens to the caregiver? This may leave the patient in the lurch. A spouse may need to modify his or her own legal documents as it is usually unwise to designate (or retain the designation of) a person with a diagnosis of dementia as another individual's POA.

Common sense rule: Don't delegate future legal responsibility to a person with dementia.

Practical Considerations in Selecting Your POA

We would like to share a few practical considerations and recommendations when selecting a POA:

1. Pick a close and trusted individual as POA.

   This may mean a close relative, but it doesn't have to be. For Medical POA, this should be a person familiar with your wishes for medical care and, most likely, who lives near you as well. Consider an individual's personality, strengths, and your relationship with this person. It makes sense to select someone who understands and is willing to carry out your medical preferences. It is also sensible to have someone who can accompany you to the doctor or visit you in the hospital, as needed. It makes no sense to appoint someone uncomfortable honoring your wishes for medical care, even if this individual is your closest relative.

2. Pick one person as primary POA, but designate alternate(s).

It is generally best to designate just one person as a primary POA and one person as secondary POA. It may also be possible and reasonable to select another person as tertiary (third in line) POA. A secondary POA may be called upon in case of death, incapacity, or any other reason the primary designee can't or won't serve as POA. Be sure and check with each individual about his or her willingness to serve in a POA role.

3. Consider separation of powers.

The same person may be granted all powers of attorney or one person may serve as Medical POA and another as general POA. Sometimes it is easiest and best to designate one person (e.g., a spouse or the only adult child who lives close to a patient) as both Medical and general POA. On the other hand, this is a great deal of responsibility and may add to caregiver burden. Depending on individual circumstances, it may work well to divide these powers. Play to the strengths of family members. For example, you might designate your daughter, who is an accountant, as your general POA, and your son, who lives close by and already helps you order medicine online, as your Medical POA.

4. Inform anyone that you designate as POA of your preferences.

The person who is to serve as your Medical POA should be aware of your medical requests, especially regarding end-of-life care and organ donation. Documents for advanced health care directives should be reviewed with your Medical POA. We recommend providing copies of medical POA and any other advanced health care directives to a patient's medical personnel (doctor, home health, nursing staff, etc.) or facility (e.g., hospital, skilled nursing, or rehabilitation unit).

Common sense rule: Pick your POA carefully.

Capacity

When One's Capacity Is in Question

When a patient's capacity to create legal documents is in doubt, a patient's attorney, doctor or a court may recommend a capacity exam conducted by a licensed psychologist or psychiatrist. Remember, capacity is specific, so the evaluation would likely focus on particular aspects, such as one's ability to designate a POA, create advanced directives, or manage one's finances. If a patient is found to have capacity for these tasks, his or her lawyer could then legally and ethically proceed in creating the appropriate documents with the patient's consent. If a patient lacks capacity for making legal decisions, the patient no longer has the option to designate a POA, nor can anyone else name a POA for such an incapacitated patient. If a patient, family, and/or other doctors dispute a professional assessment of a patient's capacity, a court may have to decide the matter.

When Capacity Is Absent

If no POA was designated prior to a patient's incapacity, life may become much more complicated for patient, family, and other caregivers. The power to make legal decisions may legally devolve to next-of-kin. Most states recognize a hierarchy of family decision-makers. If a patient is married, his or her spouse would generally be next in line to make decisions on the patient's behalf. Absent a spouse, this power would by turns usually fall to the patient's adult children, then parents (if alive), and then siblings. This may easily result in conflict, say if a patient with legal incapacity has no spouse and two or more adult children who have equal say in legal matters and don't agree on a course of action. If a patient has no family, this creates a legal vacuum. However, a patient may passively go along with any caregiver acting as a surrogate decision-maker.

How events unfold if no POA has been designated depends mightily on the involvement, cooperation, and agreement of the patient, family and other caregivers. Problems tend to arise in two specific circumstances: (1) the incapacitated individual stops cooperating with assistance or (2) evidence suggests that those providing assistance are neglecting, abusing or exploiting the incapacitated person.

In either circumstance, family may need to consider initiating guardianship proceedings. Alas, it only takes two to disagree (and one of those could be the incapacitated patient). A patient may oppose surrogate decision makers who are trying to help (or go along with surrogate decision-makers who have ill intentions). Also, it may be difficult or impossible even for a close relative (including a spouse) to perform certain legal, financial, or other functions for the patient in the absence of a designated POA. For example, a family member may be unable to withdraw funds from a bank account that is only in the patient's name—even if this money is necessary to pay for a patient's care. This may necessitate initiation of court proceedings to designate a legal guardian for the patient. This process can take time and create psychological, financial, and other costs for families who already have their hands full. In the case of suspected neglect, abuse, or exploitation, any physician or individual can report their concerns to a state adult protection agency.

Both circumstances will be discussed in more detail below, but it should be clear by now that it is far better to designate a POA in advance than to leave the door open for too many cooks, someone stirring the pot—or someone stealing it!

But what if there is no family to speak of? Unfortunately, some incapacitated individuals have no living family members or are estranged from their family. Or, perhaps all surviving family members are elderly with their own medical or other concerns and not in a position to offer assistance. The absence of family causes concern for physicians when we have patients who can no longer manage their affairs. For such patients, we recommend hiring a geriatric care manager to coordinate the assistance needed.

Or, what if family or friends are available, but a patient does not want them involved? This becomes particularly worrisome when a patient declines reasonable interventions and faces risks to health or safety. Patients with dementia may lack of awareness into their problems. Once such insight is compromised, a patient may feel that he or she doesn't need any help despite objective evidence to the contrary. Symptoms of paranoia may also impede our ability to move forward. As physicians, we can make recommendations to bring in help or move to a higher level of care, but we lack the ability to implement these changes.

Such cases call for flexibility. We might ask our patient to choose a trusted family member or friend and call the patient's designee via speakerphone with the patient present. We could discuss the situation, and ask for input and assistance (including accompanying the patient to future appointments). We can also enlist the support of a patient's primary care physician to see if he or she can intervene. A geriatric care manager may also be helpful in these circumstances. As always, we are guided by the best interests of the patient.

Guardianship

Unfortunately, situations arise where little choice remains but to file for guardianship, particularly if the ongoing health, safety, and general welfare of an individual outweigh other considerations. (Any imminent risks to a patient indicate a need for immediate medical and/or other intervention, such as contacting adult protective services.) A need for guardianship may come to pass when an individual whose capacity is in question neglects medical care and hygiene, lives in an unsafe situation, is subject to financial exploitation, overspends to the detriment of living expenses, or incurs some other significant risk (financial or otherwise) and is unable to provide for his or her safety. Maybe Mom wanders, allows strangers into her home, or leaves all of the food in the refrigerator to rot, but refuses to allow help in or to move. Perhaps a husband with dementia donates money a married couple needs to live on to questionable charities repeatedly soliciting him by telephone and mail. Sometimes families become concerned that a nonfamilial caregiver exhibits undue influence over a relative, driving a wedge between the individual and his or her family. For example, Dad has a new girlfriend who is unemployed and financially supported by him. When the family tries to meet the girlfriend or talk to Dad about the situation, the girlfriend blocks relatives from visiting or speaking to Dad on the telephone.

Most families hesitate to file for guardianship out of respect for their loved one's autonomy and fear of jeopardizing relationships. Instead, relatives may try unsuccessfully for long periods to reason with their loved one or create an amicable solution. Cost may be another concern. The applicant filing for guardianship must pay the initial filing fee in addition to the applicant's attorney fees throughout the process. Although the guardianship process can be costly, our experience is that the cost of not intervening can be greater in the end, especially when the "alleged incapacitated person" overspends, gives away their estate, or suffers financially exploitation.

Common sense rule: Guardianship is a costly, but sometimes necessary step.

Any interested party (the "applicant") can seek guardianship of another individual (the "alleged incapacitated person"). A family member often initiates this process. However, in the absence of a willing or able relative, the court may appoint an independent guardian, typically an attorney or someone from a senior services agency experienced in the management of a person's well-being and estate.

So, how does one file for guardianship? Since the specifics vary from state to state, we again recommend that you work with an attorney who practices in the state where the "alleged incapacitated person" lives. Of course, every case differs, but here is a basic overview of how the process may work:

First, the person requesting to serve as the guardian (of the person, estate or both) files an application with the probate court. States may offer an emergency guardianship track to address incapacitated persons who require immediate intervention. Then, the court will probably require a Physician Certificate (or something similar) from one or more physicians. This document asks the physician to specifically define areas of incapacity and provide supporting records (such as those related to diagnosis and evaluation of dementia). If formal neuropsychological testing has been completed, a copy should be provided to the court. The court may appoint an investigator to interview the "alleged incapacitated person," the proposed guardian, family, social services (if involved), and any other relevant party. Thorough assessment of the proposed guardian helps ensure that he or she has the alleged incapacitated person's best interests in mind. After reviewing the report filed by the investigator, the judge may (1) rule that an alternative, less restrictive option meets an individual's needs or (2) appoint an attorney ad litem to represent the alleged incapacitated person at a hearing on guardianship and set a date for this. Absent a compelling reason for exclusion, the alleged incapacitated person can attend the guardianship hearing. The judge weighs available information at the hearing and issues a ruling. In case of a finding of legal incapacity or incompetence, the judge appoints a guardian for the individual.

We encourage families to inform all relevant parties of their plan to file for guardianship. Better yet, close family members (or the equivalent) should be involved well before a decision is made. Not all family members may agree with the plan (or even with a loved one's diagnosis of dementia). Even well-meaning friends and family can create chaos when coming from different points of view, particularly those who do not see your loved one regularly and do not appreciate the level of his or her impairment.

One of the biggest concerns we hear from families is that a ne'er-do-well relative is filing for guardianship in attempts to get control of a patient's finances and that the wayward relative will somehow fool the judge into granting powers to him or her. Remember, the court investigates applicants filing for guardianship. The court can deny guardianship, even to a family member, based on relevant concerns, including financial or other abuse. If you want to be proactive, another family member can file a counter application which the court will consider alongside the original.

All guardians must provide regular reports to the court to show they are adequately managing the personal and financial affairs of their wards. The state does not compensate family and friends who serve as guardians, but the judge can allocate payment for a court-appointed guardian out of the patient's estate.

Common sense rule: Putting legal powers in place in advance best prevents the need for guardianship.

Abuse and Neglect

It becomes necessary to contact the authorities when we are concerned about a patient's immediate safety, and/or if we suspect our patient is being neglected, abused or exploited by a third party. Every state has an agency designated to investigate such allegations. For simplicity, we refer to this as Adult Protective Services (APS) although the name and scope may vary by state. You can locate the name and other information on a state's official Website. Any interested party—not just physicians—can file a report with APS. Such an agency may visit the individual's home to assess the condition of the person and his/her environment; interview the client, as well as relatives, doctors, and other relevant parties, and then make recommendations.

Bear in mind that adult protection agencies work differently than child protection agencies. Adult agencies seek to maintain the autonomy of the individual whenever possible by connecting their client with community resources. They lack legal power to force a client to accept services. And, although APS does not charge to investigate, it also doesn't cover the expense of recommended services. However, APS does partner with government and community agencies that provide free, discounted, and/or subsidized services to the adult population.

APS may only remove someone from his or her home if its assessment indicates that the person is in imminent danger. Be advised that the imminent danger standard is quite high so as to protect the rights of the individual. Relatives and/or other concerned parties may assess the situation quite differently and become frustrated that APS did not force an intervention. If APS cannot find a workable solution to the situation, it may recommend guardianship and try to find a suitable family member to serve in this role. If none is willing, available, or appropriate, APS may file for a court-appointed guardian.

Advanced Health Directives

Finally, let us turn to the subject of advanced health directives. These will also be discussed in the Chap. 16: Looking Ahead. A few specific directives deserve mention:

Do Not Resuscitate (DNR) Directive. Doctors usually just refer to this as a "DNR order." It indicates that resuscitation is not to be performed on a patient whose heart or breathing stops. A person with capacity can make this. In the case of an incapacitated patient, a DNR directive may be put in place based on the decision of a Medical POA, a medical condition meeting terms of a patient's living will, and/or family input, as available and appropriate.

If a DNR directive is appropriate for a patient, it is important to make this clear. Hospitals often prominently display such directives on or about the patient and chart. A sign indicating "DNR" may be posted prominently, perhaps even over a patient's bed, or a patient may wear a special "DNR" wristband.

Out of Hospital Do Not Resuscitate (Out of Hospital DNR). This directive would apply anyplace outside of the hospital. Typically, with this directive, family or staff would not call emergency medical services (EMS) or try to administer cardiopulmonary resuscitation (CPR).

A special out-of-hospital DNR form may be required which also requires a physician's signature, so check with the patient's doctor and state requirements. Many states have DNR forms and related information available online. Determine what your state requires in terms of documentation and whether your state emergency responders recognize wristband identification. Even outside the hospital, a DNR wristband may be warranted.

Do Not Hospitalize. This directive states that a patient should not be hospitalized (and this may include evaluation in an emergency department) for any reason. Since many facilities have official or unofficial policies regarding what symptoms, illnesses, or injuries indicate that a patient should be transported to the hospital, this directive can be used to prevent repeated hospital/emergency department visits for those in advanced stages of illness.

Whether in a hospital or not, medical responders may be obligated to try and resuscitate a patient in the absence of legally acceptable documentation of DNR status (which might include paperwork and/or a wristband). A family member's verbal say-so is not enough. Therefore, keep a copy of such forms readily accessible. Carry them with you. Keep them by a loved one's bedside and in entryways at home. Also provide these to a patient's preferred hospital and any facility to which the patient is admitted.

Common sense rule: Advanced health directives are only as good as those who know about them.

In the absence of an advanced health directive, you are leaving it to someone else to make an educated guess about what you want and this may not be the person you would choose (or who wants to wear this mantle). The so-called "surrogate decision maker" is typically determined by a legally designated hierarchy. For example, if you are incapacitated and lack both advanced directives and a Medical POA, the medical team will look to your legal spouse to make decisions. Without a legally recognized spouse, such decision-making powers typically fall to an adult child (or children). And so on.

Uncertainty regarding a patient's requests can lead to additional emotional turmoil for relatives. Keep this in mind, especially when choosing a Medical POA: Even when your wishes are known, some family members will have difficulty carrying them out based on their own personal beliefs. Speaking frankly, some individuals cannot accept the burden of making the decision to terminate your care, even if they feel that is what you would want. And, absent advanced directives from a patient, many hospitals and doctors may feel obligated to continue care if any family member opposes terminating it. This really is a case in which choosing not to decide is still making a choice—and potentially a very bad one for you—and your family for all of the reasons noted above.

Common sense rule: Advanced health directives may help families as well as patients.

Summary

When it comes to legal matters relating to dementia, seek the advice of an attorney, particularly one specializing in areas of elder law, estate, and guardianship. Everyone, including patients with dementia and their caregivers, should put their legal affairs in order sooner rather than later. Only an individual with the cognitive capacity to do so may prepare such documents as a will, advanced health care directives, and Medical and other powers of attorney. No one can complete such documents for another. A person may make these powers effective immediately or designate them as durable, effective contingent upon incapacity or other factors. Such preparation, as well as other options, may help avoid an expensive, emotionally trying, and time-consuming guardianship process.

Common Sense Rules

- Consult an attorney for legal advice.
- Consider an attorney's specialty and experience regarding legal issues in dementia.
- Someone with dementia is not automatically incapacitated.
- Only you can designate your POA.
- Everyone should get their legal affairs in order and make end-of-life wishes known.
- Don't delegate future legal responsibility to a patient with dementia.
- Pick your POA carefully.
- Guardianship is a costly, but sometimes necessary step.
- Putting legal powers in place in advance best prevents the need for guardianship.
- Advanced health directives are only as good as those who know about them.
- Advanced health directives may help families as well as patients.

Websites

National Academy of Elder Law Attorneys: www.naela.org
Alzheimer's Association Legal Plans brochure: www.alz.org
National Center on Elder Abuse, US Administration on Aging: www.ncea.aoa.gov

References

1. Legal plans: assisting the person with dementia in planning for the future. http://www.alz.org/
   national/documents/brochure_legalplans.pdf. Accessed 17 April 2011.
2. Etchells E, Sharpe G, Elliott C, Singer PA. Bioethics for clinicians: capacity. CMAJ.
   1996;155(6):657–61.

Chapter 15
Selecting Level of Care

Dig the well before you are thirsty.

—Chinese proverb

Introduction

In our experience, when it comes to caring for a loved one with dementia, families tend to delay getting help. Many understandable reasons underlie this inaction, including unawareness of a relative's situation, some degree of denial regarding a loved one's illness (or its extent and consequences), guilt or shame related to asking family members or outsiders for help, depression or helplessness on the part of a caregiver, anxiety over real or perceived separation from someone very dear, as well as cost. However, such inaction often works to the detriment of our patients and families (for example, if police are repeatedly called to look for a patient with dementia who wanders from home). It's almost never too early to engage more help. And, doing so might prevent—or at least postpone—the need for a move. So, if it has crossed your mind to get additional help for yourself or another family caregiver (or to move a loved one with dementia), it's probably past time. Your friends, family, doctors, and others most likely already know and perhaps even have told you as much—you just might not have been ready to hear it.

Many families we have worked with delay such intervention, all too often waiting until a crisis situation decides the matter for them. We have frequently observed this to be the case for obviously overburdened spousal caregivers—often ignoring the medical advice of doctors and the frantic pleas of concerned family members. Unfortunately, this refusal or delaying tactic often backfires, creating a crisis situation in which the patient or caregiver requires hospitalization and an urgent decision regarding the patient's care must be made. Remember, from Chapter 7 that a loved one will only do as well as his or her caregiver is doing. The patient may require transfer to a facility quickly chosen from a limited number of immediately available

A.M. Lipton and C.D. Marshall, *The Common Sense Guide to Dementia for Clinicians and Caregivers*, DOI 10.1007/978-1-4614-4163-2_15, © Springer Science+Business Media, LLC 2013

options. Later, after such a move has been made, a patient's family may have time to more carefully consider other possibilities better suited to individual circumstances and decide to move their loved one again. Multiple moves may incur additional time, cost, and turmoil for the patient and his or her relatives. Another untoward possibility is that a patient can no longer move (e.g., due to advanced illness), and a family is stuck paying and dealing with a living situation that they would not have chosen for their loved one in an ideal state of affairs.

Moving is hard for everyone, but particularly so for patients with dementia. Therefore, when such a transition becomes necessary, it should be made with a maximum of preparation and a minimum of disruption. Regularly review the changing needs of a loved one with dementia and his or her primary caregiver with family and health care providers. Avoid relying solely on the recommendation of staff at a residential care community, as they may have a vested interest in having your loved one move to or stay in their facility at a particular level of care (e.g., if the patient resides in assisted living and the facility lacks memory care — or availability in such a unit). We have also seen facility staffs develop such a loving attachment to a patient that they have difficulty letting him or her go. Engaging additional caregiving assistance and/or moving a patient with dementia to a residential care community sooner rather than later may actually better the chance of preserving such a patient's independence. We will explain this more later in this chapter, along with how to assess the caregiving needs of a loved one with dementia, types of caregiving assistance, and residential care options.

Common sense rule: Engage help early and often.

Assessment of Caregiving Needs in Dementia

Higher Level of Care

For the purpose of this book, a higher level of care simply means that your loved one needs more assistance and/or supervision than he or she is currently receiving. This can apply to someone living at home alone who needs family to step in to help with medication and bills. It can also apply to someone who lives in an assisted living facility who now requires memory care.

Needs Assessment

Often, a doctor, patient, and family can work together to determine the care needs of an individual with dementia and how best to meet these requirements. However, if a professional in-home evaluation of a patient's caregiving needs is desired, this may be obtained by hiring a geriatric care manager, who typically performs an extensive in-home evaluation, identifies patient needs, and makes recommendations for securing care. Since this is not a medical service, Medicare and other medical insurance don't cover the cost. If a patient has long-term care insurance, it is worthwhile checking with the company to see if a similar assessment is covered by such a policy.

Informal (Familial) Assessment

We may call this assessment "informal," but it is also invaluable. And, nothing can replace a family's knowledge of a loved one. Sometimes this is all that is needed in terms of an in-home "assessment" (in conjunction with a professional medical evaluation in a doctor's office). However, sometimes a family caregiver or doctor may need more information to go on, and a relative may be asked to monitor a patient's behavior and function more closely.

It may be fairly straightforward for a spouse or other family members who live with a loved one with dementia to identify the individual's strengths and weaknesses. But it is not always easy due to emotional factors and the gradual onset of dementia (which can tend to "sneak up" on a patient and family, especially those who are closest to the patient). Moreover, additional vigilance is usually warranted for someone who lives alone and may lack awareness or remembrance of any problems. Remember, dementia usually begins with loss of insight and awareness into one's own deficits or at least the extent and consequences of these. The person with dementia is unlikely to bring problems to your attention. If you know (or suspect) that your loved one has dementia, now is the time to look around.

Here are some signs that a loved one living alone may need a higher level of care:

- Missed or incorrectly taken medications
- Police or senior services being called out to the home (especially more than once)
- Wandering or becoming lost while walking, driving, or taking public transport
- Inability to maintain personal safety (falls, leaving stove on, not locking doors, letting strangers in, etc.)
- Inability to protect self from exploitation (giving money to phone or mail solicitors, etc.)
- Unsafe driving, including unexplained collisions or dings and dents on a car
- Evidence that your loved one is missing meals
- A refrigerator containing little or no food, significant amounts of spoiled food, or inappropriate quantities of food items (such as multiple gallons of milk and heads of lettuce, but no other food)
- Loss of attention to hygiene, especially changes in an individual's usual habits (e.g., a woman who has had a standing weekly beauty appointment for decades, who has now stopped going to her usual salon)
- Bills paid late, more than once, or not at all
- Reduced or minimal activity or poor social engagement
- Presence of anxiety, angst, or frustration in daily activities

In the case of most patients with dementia who live alone, the patient is elderly and one or more of the patient's grown children must typically step in and take responsibility. Therefore, we direct this section to them. First, look Dad over. Is he bathing regularly? Has Mom's house gone from spotless to messy? Open the refrigerator and see whether Dad is buying groceries. Check a few expiration dates. Does anything look spoiled? Are there dishes in the dishwasher or sink to indicate Dad is eating regularly? Go through the bills and checkbook with him or her. Look through Mom's medications. Check quantities and dates on labels. No one likes someone snooping around or checking up on them. So, either enlist the cooperation of your parents and appeal to their needs ("Mom, I'd like to help you order your medications online." "Dad, I'd like to help you with your finances/online banking and/or change some of your bills to direct withdrawal.") or at least do not make a big production out of monitoring the situation. To avoid familial conflict, speak beforehand to any other relevant parties (e.g., other grown children) about their observations and enlist their cooperation, help, and insights.

Common sense rule: Be vigilant to identify problems.

Caregiving Options in Dementia

The remainder of this chapter covers various options for care at home and away. The latter not surprisingly includes long-term residential care, but also suggests several alternatives to a permanent move, including day programs and respite care. With the exception of home health care, Medicare does not cover any of these services, as of the writing of this book. Veterans' benefits (which may extend to spouses of veterans in some cases) and Medicaid or certain state programs may cover some of these services. Long-term care insurance often does cover such services. In our experience, families often delay exploring such benefits and it is a mistake to do so. One of the most important things that a diagnosis of dementia allows a patient and family to do is future planning. Finding out what a patient's benefits are early on and utilizing them as and when appropriate is one of the most important things that you can do as a family caregiver and may make the difference between a loved one staying at home or moving away.

Common sense rule: Identify caregiving options and benefits as soon as possible.

The challenge we give you going forward is to open your mind to the idea that, for patients with dementia and their caregivers, maintaining independence in important aspects of life may mean not trying to go it alone in all of them. In dementia, the brain can become overwhelmed by all the tasks before it. Introducing some level of assistance frees the brain to function better. A small amount of intervention may mean the difference between your loved one struggling to perform daily activities or thriving in a more social environment. A common misconception endures that the only choice is home or nursing home. Fortunately, many, many other options exist, and a little research, discussion, and planning with family, doctors, and others go a long way in finding the best of these. Aim to find the level of care allowing your loved one to function at his or her highest level—and adapt as necessary.

Family, Friends, and Neighbors

As noted in the previous section, you should regularly monitor a loved one with dementia for difficulty in daily functioning since he or she is unlikely to fully recognize these problems, especially as they progress. Family, friends, and/or neighbors can serve as tremendous assets in identifying such difficulties and assisting with everyday tasks including bill paying, grocery shopping, and medication reminders.

We encourage a team approach in dementia. Whenever possible include your loved one and other family members. Come up with a family plan of care and arrange regular meetings (say every few months) to reappraise it. Schedule and divvy up caregiving responsibilities, playing to individual strengths, existing habit, and current needs. Make sure to help the helper by looking out for the primary caregiver and providing breaks and other support, as needed.

If you are a spousal caregiver, fill pillboxes and take medications together. If your mother has dementia, buy her a pillbox in her favorite color, sit down with her once a week, and help her load it. Offer to order medications online and/or by mail (and maybe even save money in the process—this appeals to most of our patients!).

If your loved one with dementia drives, monitor this ability by riding as a passenger at least every two weeks [1]. Review of available evidence by an American Academy of Neurology panel found that even if a patient rates himself or herself as safe, this may not be the case, whereas if a caregiver rates a patient with dementia as a marginal or unsafe driver, this is "probably useful" in identifying unsafe drivers [2]. On the other hand, if a patient with dementia rates himself or herself as safe, the preponderance of evidence showed that this is NOT helpful in identifying unsafe driving. If Dad is no longer able to drive, perhaps his lifelong golf partner doesn't mind giving him a ride to and from the course (and you should make the call to his buddy to secure a ride).

Consider ways to extend familial assistance. You might arrange Meals-on-Wheels for someone who doesn't like to cook, but make sure that food doesn't go into the refrigerator only to be forgotten and uneaten. Consider hiring a housekeeper or having an existing one come more often for someone with dementia who lives alone. Look to any social or religious organizations to which a loved one belongs for additional resources to extend familial care.

Meet with accountants, attorneys, and financial advisors to make sure that documents are up to date and financial and legal affairs are in order and in the best hands. If you will serve as a patient's Power of Attorney (POA) during any future incapacity become acquainted with aspects of the domain for which you have or will have power (see Chapter 14 for further details). For example, if you have Medical POA, familiarize yourself with Dad's medical history and doctors, create a medication list, and attend his doctors' visits with him. If you have financial POA, pick a good time to review the bank statement and pay bills together. These are just a few examples. You should be able to think of many more. Work in the best interest of your loved one by drawing on your imagination, your relationship with him or her, and other means at your disposal, including this book, other books, online resources, medical and other professionals, local and national organizations, caregiver classes, social and support groups, and, most importantly, your family and other trusted individuals.

Common sense rules:

- Be creative and cooperative in helping your loved one with dementia.
- Help the Helper.
- Make a family plan of care.

Home Health

A home health evaluation first requires the order of a physician, who has determined that a patient meets certain medical criteria to justify such assessment and care. Medicare (and other insurance coverage) for home health services has notable limitations and can be complicated and confusing even for medical professionals. It certainly bears asking whether home health may be appropriate for a loved one who doesn't drive, has significantly impaired mobility, and is mostly homebound, but don't expect insurance (other than long-term care insurance) to cover extended caregiver relief, such as in-home companions.

We have found that the general public's ideas regarding Medicare coverage for home health approach the status of urban legend. Often, when we explain that a patient doesn't meet eligibility criteria for Medicare coverage for a particular service, families counter with something along the lines of "But Aunt Judy had home health and she had someone coming in three days a week. And it was covered by Medicare."

Therefore, let's review the basics in meeting Medicare criteria (as of the writing of this book) and clear up some of these misconceptions. For Medicare coverage of home health services, a physician must assess the patient is (1) in need of intermittent, skilled care and (2) housebound. Other health insurance coverage often follows Medicare guidelines.

Skilled care requires a specially trained medical professional such as a nurse, physical therapist, occupation therapist, or speech therapist. A patient may require skilled care after surgery, hospitalization, or injury. Medicare may cover additional home health services, such as social workers and home health aides for personal care (bathing, dressing, and the like)—but only if you are simultaneously receiving skilled services. When Medicare does pay for such a home health aide, it is likely to be for a few hours a week at most and may not last beyond a few weeks. This does not meet the needs of patients requiring the assistance of in-home companions — or their family caregivers. (See the following section for more information on in-home companions.)

To justify Medicare coverage for skilled services to be provided at home, a patient must have significant challenges to leaving home for services, such as living alone and being unable to drive.

We advise against using home health services as an inappropriate or inadequate substitute for regular help and supervision. By definition, home health provides intermittent services on a short-term basis, and therefore cannot provide consistent and extended care. Home health may be a vital stop-gap measure, but it is not a long-term solution.

As doctors, we consider many factors before ordering home health services. As dementia specialists, we actually prefer our patients to have outpatient physical therapy (PT), occupational therapy (OT), or speech therapy (ST) whenever possible, because it gets them out of the house and around other people. Such outpatient services may be provided at a conveniently located clinic, hospital, or the like. This may not be bad for the caregiver either. Speaking of which, a couple of specific considerations apply for our patients with dementia receiving PT, OT, ST, or similar services and their family caregivers.

If your loved one with dementia receives PT, OT, or ST, whether at home or in another setting, you should also attend each session to learn proper techniques, be available in case of a problem during therapy (e.g., a patient with dementia becomes upset with an unfamiliar person and/or environment), help with any "homework" (exercises, etc. to be done to maintain and maximize goals of therapy), and exchange updates with the therapist. This way, you can act as a "peripheral brain" to help remind your relative of safe methods for performing daily activities, which may include such basic tasks as moving, eating, and swallowing. This may literally prevent you from breaking your back — say when you have to help your relative in getting up or down. And, it will help your loved one, too.

Medicare only pays for skilled services such as PT, OT, and ST to meet certain rehabilitation goals. Problems learning and remembering experienced by patients with dementia may limit setting and achieving such objectives. Therefore Medicare may decline further services for patients unable to participate fully or those failing to benefit from current services. Nonetheless, these therapies may significantly benefit individuals with dementia. For example, a physical therapist may provide exercise and social interaction for a patient with limited opportunities for these activities. Therefore, if insurance coverage stops, a family may consider paying out of pocket to continue such PT (or a similar service) as an integral part of a patient's routine. Sometimes we encounter patients and families with psychological barriers to paying for something that they once got "free." Beware falling into this trap. Don't deprive a loved one of beneficial services just because they aren't — or are no longer — covered by Medicare or other insurance.

Senior or Community Centers

Senior or other community centers may provide free or low-cost activities for higher functioning patients. They can offer a stimulating environment for people with dementia who have minimal cognitive or behavioral impairment. Community centers, in particular, may afford a more youthful option. Since such centers generally provide no special assistance, your loved one must be able to navigate the center and activities alone or should be accompanied by you or another responsible adult. Even if your neighborhood senior center is less than ideal, a preferred center in a neighboring municipality may be available for a membership fee. Like other activities, visits to senior or community centers should be scheduled routinely as part of a patient's daily schedule or weekly calendar. If a loved one with dementia has been active for years at a local community center, it is prudent to maintain his or her usual activity (e.g., swimming or tennis) or activities in this familiar environment for as long as is feasible, which may necessitate including the company of a family or a professional caregiver.

Common sense rule: The most expensive choice is not always the best.

Adult Day Programs (Brain Therapy)

Just like PT, OT, and ST, there is also Brain Therapy. We like to use this term to describe adult day programs (also simply called day programs). After all, dementia is a disease of the brain. So, why shouldn't we employ therapy for the brain just as we utilize PT when someone has an injury or illness affecting physical function? We also find that patients and families are much more accepting of these programs when we frame the discussion in this way. We think that such therapy represents one of the best, most economical, and, sadly, most underutilized treatments for dementia.

Unlike therapies such as PT, OT, and ST, however, Medicare does not cover the cost. Long-term care insurance policies typically pay all or a portion. Patients and families are often concerned about the price of day programs, yet these cost much less than the same number of hours of a companion (see later section on companion care) and include opportunities for group interaction and activity not possible with one-on-one care. Furthermore, having patients attend such programs while family members work may allow relatives to both keep their jobs and their loved ones at home.

Day programs offer a supervised environment with cognitively and socially stimulating activities. These might include exercise, cooking, gardening, reminiscing, reading and discussing new stories, and many, many others. They may also invite speakers, participate in volunteer projects, and offer field trips. The best programs individually tailor activities and also provide services for caregivers, such as educational opportunities, libraries, and support groups.

Such programs may be found by online searches (search terms might include adult day program, day program, memory day program, and/or memory care program along with your zip code or name of your town) as well as by contacting local and national support groups and organizations. They may be located at freestanding centers as well as religious and educational institutions and community centers. Residential memory care facilities may offer them to patients who live at home as well as their own residents. This arrangement affords an opportunity for a patient and family to become well acquainted with the staff, program, other participants, and facility environment should temporary placement (i.e., respite care) or a more permanent move be later required.

Adult day programs allow an individual with dementia to continue to reside at home or another less-restrictive level of care. For example, a man with dementia and his wife may reside in assisted living. He may attend brain therapy while she goes about her activities (or takes a nap). Without this intervention, the wife might find the caregiving burden too much and her husband might have to move to a memory care unit. This example shows how such programs can, on the one hand, maintain independence even for patients who no longer reside at home while, at the same time, keeping a family together.

Brain therapy is typically offered in half-day or full-day increments on weekdays. Like other activities of daily living (ADLs), brain therapy or visits to senior or community centers should be scheduled routinely as part of a patient's weekly calendar. We have found that our patients with dementia typically derive the most benefit from a day program if they attend at least twice a week. Such regularity emphasizes the routine and regular nature of the activity. An interval of more than a few days between visits seems too long for most patients with dementia—and their caregivers!

A patient's reluctance to attend the program may pose a barrier to participation, but this problem may often be circumvented altogether. Remember that apathy is often a prominent symptom of dementia. So, if you ask your loved one about participating in any activity, you should not expect enthusiasm. Furthermore, if he or she broke his leg, you probably wouldn't ask, "Do you want to go to PT?"; you would just bring him or her there as the doctor prescribed. We recommend following a similar "just do it" approach for brain therapy. If you need, ask the patient's physician to write a "prescription" (e.g., Brain Therapy 2–3 times/week). Including a frequency with some flexibility allows you to exercise your judgment as caregiver as to whether to have your loved one attend 2 days or 3 half-days per week. If a patient balks at the idea of brain therapy, families are often reluctant to "force" someone to go. Another option is to explain it as a senior center geared toward people with memory problems. The main point, however, is not to describe it in detail in advance, but to just get your loved one there in the same way as if he or she were going to the doctor or PT, nonchalantly making it a part of routine health maintenance.

For those participants residing at home, transportation is not typically provided by day programs. However, this should not represent an insurmountable barrier. If you work, it may be easy enough to drop a loved one off and pick him or her up on your way to and from your job. You also might carpool with relatives or with family members of other participants. If timing is an issue, particularly if it takes some time to get your loved one ready for the day, you might consider hiring a professional caregiver for an hour or two in the morning to help your loved one wake up, dress, take medications, eat breakfast, etc., and then provide transportation to the program. If transportation does pose an issue, check with the program staff for suggestions (there may be another family in the same boat as you with whom you can share driving or, if you don't drive, supervisory duties) and see if your city includes dementia as a qualifying diagnosis for its transportation programs for the disabled. You may also wish for your loved one to attend say 2 full-day sessions rather than 4 half-day sessions to minimize travel.

Family caregivers will probably want to visit the program, see the facility, and speak to the staff initially without the patient. One visit is not enough for your loved one to feel comfortable, particularly when you take into account the stress of a new environment. It is reasonable to give it a try for a set time period and reassess. We suggest that a patient attend at least two to three times a week for a month before deciding to discontinue. Like other treatments for dementia, it deserves a full, fair trial.

Brain therapy represents an economical way for a patient with dementia to get out of the house but still reside at home while giving family caregivers a break. If you don't have a program like this in your area, consider teaming with the local chapter of your Alzheimer's Association, additional community groups, and other caregivers to start one.

Sometimes caregivers feel guilty about sending their loved one to brain therapy, but this may be a way to get a patient with dementia out of the house, socially engaged, and physically and mentally active. Remember, not only might the caregiver need a breather, but the patient may need a break from the caregiver!

Common sense rule: The patient may need a break from the caregiver!

Companion Care

Companion care provides one-on-one supervision. Sometimes such professional caregivers are called in-home companions and their involvement certainly may extend patients' ability to stay in their own homes. However, companions may also be employed in environments such as hospitals, nursing facilities, assisted living, memory care units, etc. They are also sometimes called sitters, but we shy away from using this term. If this expensive form of caregiving must be employed, we prefer that such a companion does more than just sit! It is important to distinguish companion care from in-home "24-hour nursing" care. Nurses understandably command a higher hourly, but formalized nursing training is rarely needed to provide the companionship, stimulation, assistance, and supervision that dementia patients need.

Most professional caregivers are paid by the hour and many require a minimum daily commitment (e.g., 4 hours). For round-the-clock care, agencies commonly offer a weekly rate. There may be some upfront payment, but services are usually billed month to month. Depending on policy restrictions, long-term care insurance may cover this service, but Medicare (and other health insurance) does not.

Some state programs provide limited coverage for such companion services for low-income seniors; however, the wait may be lengthy, sometimes over a year. Contact your state's Department of Aging to inquire about programs and eligibility and to place your loved one's name on any waiting list.

The experience of professional caregivers varies widely. They may be hired from a companion agency or work independently. If your loved one has had a home health agency that you like, you may check with them to see if you could hire such a companion through them. Ask family, friends, and medical professionals for recommendations. Social workers are particularly helpful and knowledgeable about such agencies. Geriatric care organizations and associations can provide lists of local companion agencies. Search senior newspapers and the like as well as online, preferably by going directly to known websites and then using specific terms like in-home companion or companion care. If you do a general search for companion, you may get much more than you bargained for ....

Companion care agencies may be harder to find in rural areas, but friends or family may know of someone who may be available to hire privately and this might be someone your loved one already knows (or from a familiar family). Also try reaching out to social, religious, and community organizations, especially those for which your loved one has a connection.

If choosing between paying an agency for companions or employing an independent operator, weigh the advantages and disadvantages of each carefully. Working with an agency may necessitate rotating different individuals, but may be advantageous in providing depth of staff (as opposed to the situation you may find yourself in if you hire one companion who falls ill).

Furthermore, agencies often provide background checks, bonding, certification, and insurance for such companions, but check with the individual company. Make sure to check these factors for anyone you hire who works independently. You may want to perform your own background check as well. As you would for any service, comparison shop, get several quotes, and negotiate charges. They may be worth the cost and have enough demand for their services that they won't budge on the price, but it's always worth asking.

We recommend paying for any companion to attend the professional caregiver class through your local chapter of the Alzheimer's Association. If you hire companions through an agency and they already have caregiver training in dementia, this is a very good sign, but we still recommend this specific course.

Always interview potential candidates to find a good fit. Allow a trial period before making any long-term commitments. Keep in mind that sometimes a firmer personality may work better than a gentle one to enforce a certain level of activity. Find someone who can create a routine and not be talked out of it by the patient. A great companion just starts putting on those tennis shoes instead of asking, "Would you like to go for a walk?"

A patient with dementia may reject the idea of a companion due to the expense as well as the idea of someone coming in his or her home. Our experience is that if you address one concern, your loved one will just come up with another. We therefore recommend against prolonged explanations, but instead putting the companion in place and allowing an adjustment period. Sometimes, we and families can sell the idea in terms of help with housekeeping, transportation, and meal preparation instead of companionship and supervision. Many families refer to the companion as "the housekeeper" or "friend," and a professional caregiver experienced in dealing with patients with dementia will happily adopt this title. Likewise, we may choose wording to promote the idea that the help is being brought in for the caregiver spouse. And it's also true! Many of our dementia patients would balk at the idea that they need assistance but would readily accept "housekeeping" help for their wife with health problems. Sometimes, such caregiving assistance becomes essential to maintain the health and safety of a patient with dementia, who may be oblivious to this need due to poor insight. It is therefore crucial for families to communicate and otherwise ally themselves with companions. If you hire, supervise, and direct companions to provide necessary care, then your loved one can't "fire" them.

Respite Care

Respite care typically equates to a short-term stay (from days to weeks) at a memory care or a similar facility, such as nursing home. Although Medicare and other health insurance typically don't cover respite care, Veterans' Benefits and long-term care insurance policies often do, at least to some extent.

Respite care provides a valuable and probably underused option for patients with dementia who needs 24-hour supervision while their family caregivers are otherwise engaged. It may be utilized for medical reasons (e.g., a caregiver having surgery), family vacations (or other trips to be made without the patient), other situations in which a caregiver's attention needs to be elsewhere, or simply a much-needed break for the family caregiver.

In many circumstances, families wish to travel and it is overly burdensome or not appropriate to bring along their loved one with dementia. This may include weddings, births, or vacations. Sadly, families may also need to travel to deal with sickness or death.

In some scenarios, it may be possible to arrange respite care quickly, but, as with most dementia care situations, a little planning goes a long way. For a patient to be admitted to respite care, a doctor must complete and sign forms detailing a patient's history, examination, diagnosis, and medications, as well as orders for diet, medications, etc. Proof that a patient does not have tuberculosis (TB) may be required, necessitating a chest X-ray or a TB test (which must be placed a few days before it can be read). If a doctor's office receives blank forms on a Friday afternoon, admission that weekend is probably not feasible. Ideally, you should make preparations for respite care once dates for a planned trip or elective surgery are known. In any event, try to allow at least a few days for the facility to make arrangements and the doctor/s to complete paperwork. Follow up to ensure that the facility has indeed faxed the forms to the patient's doctor/s. We find it useful for our patients to have such paperwork completed by their primary care physician, as it typically requires information from the last physical examination. If you have a specialist managing the dementia and/or psychiatric medication, have that physician fax the last progress note detailing the current dementia medication regimen so that any discrepancies can be resolved before admission. This way, the facility has history, exam, medications, and orders pertinent to a patient's dementia as well as other medical conditions.

If you are considering respite care, utilize this opportunity to visit several facilities and become familiar with them. Then, enroll your loved one in the respite program of your choice. This allows you to "test drive" the facility in advance of any permanent placement that may later be necessary. Moreover, familiarity with the residents, staff, activities, and physical environment may later serve as a significant comfort for your loved one if placement becomes permanent, particularly if you use the same facility on several occasions or regularly. If appropriate in an individual case, respite care may be extended into permanent placement and this option may be preferable if a patient has adjusted well to the facility, is doing better there than at home, and a transition back home might be detrimental.

If you don't have a memory care unit in your area, a nursing home or a similar facility may offer respite care, but exercise caution. Staff in a general nursing facility may lack the specialized training of those working in a memory unit. However, since they often work with the elderly, they usually have some experience in working with patients with dementia. The experience and skill level can vary from individual to individual, facility to facility—and shift to shift! If you don't have other options for respite care, a nonspecialized unit may be worth a try. You might speak to the director or other administrator to find out about staff education and facility policies specific to dementia.

Furthermore, the facility may not be suitable for a patient with dementia if it is not locked or "secure" (as a memory care unit would be) and allows patients to exit without knowledge of the staff. This could obviously pose a problem for a patient who wanders, but even a patient with dementia who has never wandered before may do so in an unfamiliar environment. If a secure (locked) memory care unit is not available, a patient may need 24-hour supervision, such as is provided by in-home companion care.

Family members other than the primary caregiver can also be a wonderful (and free) source of respite care. Regardless of who is providing respite care, make sure to inform them of your loved one's typical daily routine, including (but definitely not limited to) medications. The best respite care programs offer activities akin to the brain therapy discussed above to maintain social engagement and physical and mental health.

Common sense rule: Respite care offers a temporary option to permanent placement.

Residential Care

Making Plans to Move Your Loved One

Moving is hard. Moving is even harder for those with dementia and their families. If you are even considering this step, it is worth exploring options in your community to give you time to find the right one. Nowadays, the choice is no longer limited to home or nursing home. As we discuss in this section, a variety of options exist to meet the needs of people with dementia and their families. However, many facilities have waiting lists. It's worth putting your loved one's name on the waiting list for the facility. If an apartment becomes available before you are ready, you can always defer ("Mom doesn't need to move right now, but please keep us on the waiting list."). Utilize advice of family, friends, and fellow caregivers, as well as doctors and other professionals (e.g., social workers, geriatric care managers) in identifying community resources. Most of all, visit facilities at least a few times, speak with staff, and ask questions. If you can, speak with other family members who have loved ones with dementia who live there. And, make sure to sit in on a meal and try the food!

Sadly, many such moves are precipitated by a trip to the hospital. If a patient is not safe to be discharged home alone or with family, Medicare and other health insurance will not cover additional hospital days to allow family time to find placement in an appropriate residential care facility. We have seen many families in a frenzy trying to find something workable on a tight time frame. Our advice is to move your loved one before the storm erupts rather than in the midst of it. Since one of the goals of placement is to preserve functioning, it is counterintuitive to wait until someone is in crisis.

So, don't wait until Dad bottoms out before moving him. Even if he is doing fine in his current environment, determine in advance where he will go if he needs a higher level of care. That way, your tours and research will be conducted in a non-crisis mode in which you can think clearly. If an event triggers the need to move quickly, it is much more likely for this to transpire smoothly if you have already visited and vetted a facility. It's the search that takes the time. If and when living at home is no longer an option, planning and preparation ensure that your loved one with dementia will literally be in the best place.

Common sense rules:

- Don't delay in finding a facility to best suit the needs of your loved one with dementia.
- Get on the waiting list for the facility of choice.

Independent Living

Although people who live at home may live independently, the term "independent living," in this context, refers to residing in a home or an apartment within a senior community. Residents are expected to function on their own in this environment. Local transportation may be offered via a van or a shuttle service. A meal plan in a dining hall may be purchased and offer welcome socialization. Additional social and other activities may be available. Independent living is unlikely to be covered by any type of insurance or benefits.

Independent living works best for patients with minimal deficits and/or whose families can step in to provide assistance. A candidate for independent living might need transportation, meal provision, and/or social and other activities and should be self-motivated to engage with others and participate in the programs on offer. A general rule of thumb is that if someone cannot function independently at home, he or she will not function successfully in independent living. Therefore, it is generally NOT advisable to move a patient with dementia from home to independent living as it provides no advantage. Moving to assisted living or a memory care unit usually makes much more sense. However, this is one of the most common mistakes we see from well-meaning families.

> A 73 year-old man is diagnosed with Alzheimer's disease by his family doctor. He isn't eating regularly or paying bills on time. He's missing medication and having delusions that someone is stealing from him. He's not keeping up with his hygiene or housekeeping.
>
> Worried that Dad can no longer live in his home safely, his adult children move him to an independent living apartment closer to them and take over bill-paying. His daughter loads a pillbox for him, but he continues to miss medication because he forgets to take it. And, even though the facility staff and residents go out of their way to welcome Dad and invite him to activities, he stays in his apartment all day. He has meals delivered to his room rather than eating in the dining hall. His family has noticed him to become increasingly anxious and brings him to a geriatric psychiatrist for evaluation.

This example shows that Dad needs a higher level of care than independent living. Perhaps he is overwhelmed by trying to find his way in a new place and therefore retreating to his apartment. Increased supervision is essential for his general health and well-being, including ensuring that his medications are administered correctly, addressing his anxiety and increasing his activity level. In this situation, Dad would most likely need to move yet again, either to assisted living or memory care. The lesson here is to avoid a move that won't help and might harm.

Common sense rules:

- Independent living is not a good option for patients with dementia having problems living at home.
- Set a patient up for success. Don't set a patient up for failure.

Assisted Living

Most patients and families find it surprising that the lowest levels of assisted living do not include much more beyond independent living than meal service. Some facilities offer an inclusive package pricing scheme. However, in most cases, you pay a base price for assisted living to which additional services can be purchased à la carte. These options may include:

1. Medication reminders or administration
2. Assistance with ADLs, such as bathing and dressing
3. Assistance with household chores (housekeeping, laundry service)

In assisted living lingo, you may hear about different "levels" of care which are attached to different price points. Higher levels include the most services and are higher priced. Larger facilities may separate levels of care by floors or wings. Residents on the third floor may be receiving full services while those on the first floor receive the least. Medicare and other types of health insurance do not pay for assisted living, but Veterans' Benefits or a long-term-care insurance policy may cover all or a portion of the cost. Veterans may also have access to Veterans' Affairs assisted living facilities.

The advantage of assisted living is that residents can maintain their independence with appropriate services in place. There is a level of supervision built in as staff checks on each resident's welfare daily. There is usually a licensed vocational nurse (LVN) on site, but this may be limited to daytime hours. Make sure to visit the facility, preferably on a few occasions at a few different times of day (e.g., meal time, activity time) and days of the week.

Here are some questions you might ask about assisted living:

What is included in the base price?

Is an upfront fee or long-term commitment required?

Does the facility have a social worker or an administrator who could help in determining whether your loved one might qualify for Veterans' or other benefits that might defray the cost?

What are the additional care options available (e.g., medication administration, assistance with ADLs, housekeeping) and how much do they cost?

Is moving within the facility (or out of it) necessary if a resident needs more care?

What activities are available?

What happens if a patient doesn't show up to a meal or an activity? (i.e., Does a staff member knock on the resident's door and encourage attendance or not?)

Is one or more nurse on site?

What are the nurses' hours?

Does the facility procure medications or does the family need to do this for a patient? (If the facility obtains these, it takes the onus off the caregiver, but you might compare prices to see if the cost is worth it.)

Does the facility have a physician available to see patients on site?

Does the physician have a geriatric psychiatrist available to see patients on site?

How does the move-in process work and does the facility have any suggestions or offer help to ease the transition?

Are pets allowed (important to know if the patient has a pet or allergies)?

When it is necessary for patients with dementia to move because they are no longer able to safely live at home, it is generally not a good idea to ask if they "want to." They most likely won't agree. After all, you probably don't "want" your loved one to move from home either, although it may be a necessary step. If it is required for a patient's safety and well-being, it works well for families to meet and choose a facility and make the move as seamless as possible, gently encouraging the patient's cooperation. The involvement of someone with dementia depends on each individual case and multiple factors, including the severity of cognitive deficits, incapacity, current living situation, and health status. Check with your loved one's doctors and the facility for additional information and advice on how best to do this in your situation. Some patients may be able to visit two or three facilities with a family member and help choose one. Patients with such severe dementia that family members must handle all details and move them in with little or no notice may be better suited for memory assisted living or a memory care unit as is discussed in the following section.

Common sense rule: Ask questions.

Memory Assisted Living/Memory Care/Alzheimer's Unit

Memory care goes by many names. In this section we discuss two main types: Memory assisted living and Memory care (or Alzheimer's) units. A program with memory or Alzheimer's in its name tends to indicate a higher level of care than assisted living as well as secure (locked) units. However, please note that these terms are not standardized. You need to do careful research, visit facilities, and ask questions to find the right level of care for your loved one. Don't judge a program by its title (or its décor). To avoid confusion with "Memory assisted living," non-memory assisted living will be referred to as "traditional assisted living" for the remainder of this chapter. Memory assisted living is usually more expensive than traditional assisted living, and memory care tends to cost the most of all forms of residential care. Like their traditional counterpart, memory assisted living and other types of memory care are not covered by Medicare and other types of health insurance. Veterans' Benefits or a long-term-care insurance policy may cover all or a portion of the cost.

Some facilities will offer a reduced rate for shared rooms or suites in which your loved one has a roommate. Unfortunately, the presence of a stranger in the room is not always well received. Patients may try to physically remove the "intruder." However, shared rooms may work for individuals with dementia who are generally neither agitated nor paranoid and either like having someone to talk to or do not pay much attention to a roommate.

Memory assisted living splits the difference between assisted living and memory care. Some facilities may offer memory-assisted living as the highest level of traditional assisted living. Other facilities may offer memory assisted living as the lowest level of memory care. Other facilities may offer memory assisted living exclusively.

Staffs at a memory assisted living program tend to be more proactive than those working in traditional assisted living in encouraging patients to participate in activities. Medication administration, housekeeping, and assistance with ADLs should be included in the price of memory assisted living since a patient who is forgetful might be expected to have difficulty performing these tasks independently.

Memory assisted living works best for those with moderate-to-severe dementia who cooperate with their care and lack significant behavioral issues. Residents tend to be socially engaged and able to participate in activities. The residential unit may have ample space to move about, but all doors leaving the unit will be locked to prevent a resident from leaving unattended. Family members and guests will use a code to enter and exit.

Memory (or Alzheimer's) care units can better accommodate patients with behavioral issues, such as resistance to care, combativeness, and wandering. This level also caters to individuals who need the maximum assistance with ADLs. The daily routine is structured and the unit is secure, although many facilities also offer protected freedom to roam in enclosed courtyards or walkways.

Common sense rule: Don't judge a program by its title (or its décor).

When Is the Time for Memory Care?

We are often baffled when a family decides to move a loved one with significant cognitive and/or behavioral deficits into traditional assisted living despite obvious signs indicating a need for memory care. Again, we caution you not to set your loved one up for failure. Consult with a patient's doctors to assess the best level of care. Do not rely solely on the advice of facility personnel for reasons discussed previously. Likewise, do not let your emotions overwhelm your decision-making abilities. We recommend you rely on the following criteria.

Memory assisted living or memory care should be considered if your loved one with dementia has one or more of the following signs or symptoms:

- Wandering
- Physical aggression
- Verbal altercations
- Agitation
- Socially inappropriate behavior (such as disrobing)
- Persistent irritability
- Other significant behavioral problems
- Psychosis with hallucinations, delusions, and/or paranoia
- Inattention to or difficulty with basic hygiene
- Resistance to necessary assistance with bathing and incontinence care
- Significant social isolation

When deciding on moving a loved one with dementia, families tend to get stuck in three areas:

1. Not convinced the time to move is now.
2. Thinking your loved one is not as impaired as the other residents.
3. Worrying your loved one will be miserable if moved.

These issues often come into play for any move for a loved one with dementia, but particularly arise when time comes for memory care. Let us tackle these concerns one by one.

1. Not convinced the time to move is now.

    The first category includes families who are "waiting for a sign." They believe that things may not be going well, but are not that bad. It is helpful to have reasonable indication that something needs to change. However, some families minimize signs obvious to others and are truly awaiting a crisis. Many moves to memory care arise from a crisis situation—such as police involvement or a psychiatric hospitalization. Our experience is that it never works well to wait until things get that bad to make a move.

    The point of moving someone with dementia is stabilization. It's easier to calm a less than ideal situation than a disastrous one. The name of the game in this illness is slowing decline. If we wait for major deterioration to trigger a move, we've already lost ground.

2. Thinking your loved one is not as impaired as the other residents.

    Next, let us address the level of impairment. If you note large discrepancies between the level at which your loved one is functioning compared to other residents in memory care, you could try to find a facility that fits more with the memory assisted living model described above. However, we commonly find that families perceive a big difference when there isn't one for two major reasons. First, you've witnessed your loved one's decline over years. When you walk into a memory care facility, you are seeing a snapshot of someone else's loved one. You may perceive your loved one's deficits as milder because the changes are subtle over time. This works similarly to watching children grow. You may not see much alteration over 6–12 months, whereas friends and family who visit once or twice a year may be astonished at the amount of change. Secondly, when it comes to dementia, we are all at risk for some level of denial which makes it challenging to accurately assess a loved one's abilities.

3. Worrying your loved one will be miserable if moved.

    Finally, will your loved one be miserable? The answer is probably not. The structure, socialization, assistance, and activities provided often increase a resident's level of functioning and decrease mood, anxiety, and behavioral issues. Patients who have lost weight due to forgetting meals may gain back pounds. However, be prepared for the first few days or weeks to be challenging. Allow time for adjustment for your loved one, yourself, and other family members. You may even wish to refrain from visiting for the first few days to allow your loved one to settle in. Your loved one may be angry or demand to leave. This may lead to repeated phone calls or arguing during visits. To understand how difficult moving is for a patient with dementia, imagine if you found yourself confused and in an unfamiliar place. Now imagine that you don't speak the language. Explanations are not going to be nearly as helpful as hugs and other reassurance. These behaviors generally improve with time. Facility staffs will assist and advise you in the transition and, as previously noted, it's best to coordinate with them even prior to the move.

Common sense rule: Know signs indicating the need for supervised and secure living.

Different Levels of Care/Facilities That Offer Multiple Levels of Care

We often recommend that families consider communities with different levels of care for several reasons. One is the ability for patients to stay in the same facility as needs change. This may be particularly advantageous for a patient living with a spouse, partner, or other family member.

For example, let's say that Mom has dementia while Dad is cognitively intact but needs day-to-day help with Mom. Mom and Dad want to live together. First, look for a facility that offers different levels of care. You have many options. For couples who want to stay together in one apartment, typically we lean toward the level of care more fitting to Mom since she needs more services. This is most compelling when Mom needs a secure (locked) environment or has behavioral issues. But Dad may balk at living with people with significant impairment. So Dad may choose to live in an independent living apartment so that he can be more socially and cognitively engaged with his peers, while Mom lives in a memory care unit in the same facility. Because he's on the same campus, he can regularly visit and eat meals with his wife. However, if Mom lacks wandering or behavioral issues, they could try splitting the difference in levels of care needed and reside in assisted living together. Ask the facility director if Mom can attend the memory care activities if that would be beneficial to her (and maybe a break for Dad). And, if one option does not work out as intended, a facility with different levels of care allows you to try others.

Although we find institutions with multiple levels of care to have many benefits, one disadvantage that we have regularly encountered is that patients seem to stay in one of the lower levels of care much longer than is appropriate. You may need to assert the need for your loved one to move to memory care. Consult with your loved one's doctors and get their help in advocating for such a move if it is warranted. If space in that facility's memory assisted living or memory care unit is not available, work with the facility staff to determine options to meet your loved one's needs or even look outside the facility, if needs be.

This industry is adapting to the growing needs of the aging population. Some independent living communities partner with or allow home health and companion agencies to provide on-site services to their residents. And, frankly speaking, traditional assisted living facilities manage a large number of dementia patients. The 2009 Overview of Assisted Living, which collects data from assisted living and senior housing agencies, estimates that over a third of all traditional assisted living residents have a dementia diagnosis [3]. Empirical studies have found that 45–67 % of traditional assisted living residents have some level of dementia [4, 5]. Over the last few years, we have seen more and more assisted living communities allow their residents, in the absence of behavior or safety issues, to stay in assisted living despite significant cognitive impairment. We can certainly appreciate the good intentions of allowing patients with dementia to stay in a familiar environment; however, an appropriate level of care should not be inadvertently avoided or delayed. The right level of care is best for patients with dementia as well as for all of their caregivers, family, and professional caregivers alike.

Common sense rules:

- Consider facilities that offer multiple levels of care.
- Make the move to a higher level of care as and when needed.

Residential Care Home/Personal Care Home

Some individuals and families may prefer the smaller, homelike environment of houses in residential areas staffed with professional caregivers (usually with at least one nurse on-site during the day and/or available by phone). These are known as residential care homes. One advantage is the homey feel. Residential care homes may work better than large nursing facilities for some patients by providing a more "person-centered" level of care [6]. They offer increased flexibility for individual needs, e.g., for a patient who has a special pet, who smokes, or who becomes agitated by the presence of many people. The latter category may include someone with dementia who has "always been a loner," but it also includes patients with dementia who now can't or won't engage in social activities offered by larger communities. The resident's day is traditionally less structured which may also work well for patients who have unusual sleep–wake patterns.

Because there are fewer residents in such homes, there are also usually fewer caregivers, although the staff:patient ratio is often far better than that of large facilities. The caution is to make sure that the available personnel can manage any medical and behavioral issues pertinent to your loved one. Cost and proximity may also come into play in deciding whether this environment works well. And, like assisted living and memory care, Medicare and other health insurance doesn't cover the cost of a residential care home. Long-term-care insurance might.

Nursing Home/Skilled Nursing Facility

Although nursing home care is listed at the end of our facility list, it is not meant to imply that this is a higher level of care than memory care or that all patients will eventually go to a nursing home. Patients with dementia can stay in assisted living or memory care through their last days unless money to pay for such care runs out or medical needs require a higher level of nursing.

A skilled nursing facility (SNF, often pronounced "sniff," also known as a skilled nursing unit or SNU) may be part of a nursing home, hospital, or other care institution. Medicare may cover a few days or weeks of skilled nursing if a patient meets several conditions, including a qualifying hospitalization (usually at least a few days). It is important to know that a hospital physician cannot prolong a hospital stay for the sole purpose of meeting this requirement. A patient must also have the ability to participate and benefit from the services offered, which may include physical, occupation, and speech therapy, as well as nursing care. This can be an issue when dementia interferes with a person's ability to participate — such as when your loved one is unable to follow a therapist's instructions or refuses to participate.

If your loved one with dementia is hospitalized for any reason, ask to speak with a social worker and check about your loved one's eligibility for skilled nursing upon discharge from the hospital. If you have selected a facility for placement or your loved one already resides in such a facility, that institution may have its own SNF or SNU that can be utilized. A social worker can help arrange skilled nursing for an eligible patient. The requirements for Medicare to pay for inpatient rehabilitation care are similar but even more stringent. If a patient is not eligible for skilled nursing, home health services may be an option, not only for patients who live at home, but also for those in independent, assisted, or memory care. For example, a patient who lives in an Alzheimer's unit might be eligible for Medicare coverage for physical therapy. The hospital social worker can help you sort this out.

A long-term-care insurance policy may alleviate some or all of the cost of nursing home care. Medicare and other health insurance do not cover long-term care in nursing facilities. However, Medicaid, which provides assistance to low-income individuals, may cover nursing home costs. Be aware that not all nursing homes accept Medicaid. Those that do may limit the number of beds that are available for Medicaid recipients. When a Medicaid bed becomes available in a facility, preference is typically given to existing residents who exhausted their funds while paying for their care at that facility. Patients may have no (or very limited) choice of facility and/or have to wait for a bed to become available. Consult an attorney as the rules and regulations, particularly regarding assets, are complicated and vary from state to state. Since Medicaid is administered by the state in which your loved one resides, it is important to consult with an attorney in that state, preferably one who specializes in Medicaid eligibility and benefits and, perhaps, an elder law attorney. Patients and families often express reluctance to take on the cost of attorney consultation, particularly since they are considering Medicaid in the first place due to limited financial resources. However, the feedback we have received from families consistently supports the idea that assistance is needed to navigate the Medicaid application process.

Social workers may also be of considerable help. They may be contracted privately, but their services may be covered as part of hospitalization, home health, Veterans' benefits, or residence at a facility.

Hospice

Many people think of Hospice in the context of cancer, but Hospice can offer significant help to patients with dementia at the end of life and their families. Did you know that Hospice can provide additional nursing and medical care? Pay for prescription medications? Offer social and spiritual services to the family as well as the patient?

Medicare has specific criteria for Hospice eligibility. A diagnosis of dementia ALONE is not enough. A patient must meet other criteria, such as substantial weight loss, total bowel and bladder incontinence, and loss of mobility (e.g., a patient who was walking, who is now confined to bed, or has to use a wheelchair). If you notice such changes in your loved one with dementia, it is important to bring them to the attention of a doctor and to request a Hospice evaluation because a physician must also certify that a patient has 6 months or fewer to live. If you aren't sure, remember—an evaluation is just an evaluation. You have no obligation to accept Hospice services.

Hospice has served as an invaluable asset in the care of our patients and their families which is why we are generally inclined to order or concur with a Hospice evaluation for our patients with severe dementia. Dementia, after all, is ultimately a terminal illness. However, many families are significantly unnerved by the idea, because they have the "six months to live" definition firmly ingrained in their minds. Hospice forces us to address end-of-life issues, which often elicits resistance, anger, sadness, and fear. Some family members may feel like they've just been informed of imminent death at the mere mention of the word Hospice. Relatives may have watched a slow decline and just don't see any acute change. Families may also fear that Hospice will come in, stop all of a loved one's medication, and actually hasten death. In reality, we have found Hospice teams to be sensitive and receptive to our suggestions as dementia specialists regarding our patients' medications and other needs. We have also seen case after case which goes to show that Hospice should be used sooner rather than later. A Hospice team usually spends a great deal of time and effort working with patients and families. The amount of help that they can provide is related to the amount of time that they are able to identify needs and plan and provide services. If Hospice is called for in the last few days of a patient's life, they have little chance to become acquainted with the patient and family and address any issues, whereas if they are involved for weeks or months, they can meet a multitude of medical, nursing, social, spiritual, and other needs.

Common sense rule: Think of Hospice sooner rather than later.

Choosing a Facility

In making this important choice, consider Program, Proximity, and Price. Most families will have to balance these factors in making their selection.

Program refers to the type of facility, level of care, and activities and assistance offered. Now that you know the different types of facility, you are better equipped to look for the right one. You do not have to tour ten facilities. You can start with asking friends and other caregivers, professionals (doctor, social worker, geriatric care manager, etc.), online searches, and associations for patients and caregivers. Utilize a variety of Web- and non-Web-based resources to obtain the fullest picture of what is available in your community. Check Websites for state agencies responsible for inspection, regulation, certification, and licensing. A number of for-profit Websites may only show facilities and other agencies that advertise with them. These can still be very helpful resources; just consider the source and any potential bias. Also look at individual facility Websites.

Narrow your search to three or so places to tour. Speak with administration and staff, but also talk with residents and family members about their experience. Ask for a schedule and a menu. Drop by unannounced. Eat the food. Observe the residents and activities. Also consider whether it makes sense to move your loved one from facility to facility as she needs higher levels of care. Even if Mom doesn't need much care now, consider a facility that has several levels of care so that she can remain in the same facility. This is the idea of "aging in place." Your loved one may have to eventually move to another floor, wing, or building in the complex, but that will generally be much easier than going to a new facility.

When it comes to *Proximity*, think of the old real estate axiom, "location, location, location." The location should be directed by factors such as proximity to the family member/s (or other individual/s) who will visit most often and meaningful activities (such as clubs, social group, or religious institutions). An otherwise nice facility may not be the best choice if the closest family member lives so far away as to make visiting difficult. Be creative in problem solving. Consider moving your loved one to a facility close to beloved people and activities or arrange transportation through the facility, friends, family, or neighbors to allow interaction and participation as long as feasible and experienced positively by your loved one.

Price. It is important to obtain the right level of care for a loved one, while ensuring that their means are not exhausted. Meet and communicate early and often with involved family members and similarly involved parties to avoid misunderstandings and to discuss options and preferences. Get information from a facility in writing. Consider carefully before signing documents. If you're not sure, sleep on it. You may also try to negotiate the price, especially raising any extenuating circumstances, such as moving two parents to the same facility. As with any major financial or real estate transaction, consider advice from a financial planner and/or attorney. Consider hiring a social worker or a geriatric care manager for the informative assessments they may provide. Veterans and surviving spouses may be eligible for various levels of assistance, including the help of a social worker. Contact your local Veterans' Administration for eligibility.

And, finally, consult with a patient's physicians regarding predicted disease duration and life expectancy. We often hear something along these lines:

> I know memory care would be good for Dad, but he really can't afford it. We talked to Dad's financial advisor. The advisor told us Dad would run out of money in three years if he moved to that level of care.

Since we're all living longer, it is challenging to plan for the future. So this is how we look at it. Because no one has a crystal ball, we simply have to weigh the benefits and risks to the best of our understanding. Will Dad's money likely last him to the end of his life if he stays where he is? If the answer is yes or probably, there is more to think about because we run the risk of depleting his funds with the move. However, if Dad is 85 years old with severe dementia and multiple medical problems, the move may be worth the risk because his predicted life expectancy may only be a couple of years.

However, if Dad will likely outlive his savings, it surprisingly makes the decision easier. Unless family assumes Dad's care or steps in with additional funding, Dad is heading toward needing Medicaid which could cover nursing home care. Since Dad would benefit from memory care, we would argue that it is better for Dad to spend his money on memory care during the years he is most aware and can benefit most from this level of care. This way, if he lives long enough that he runs out of money, his dementia may be so far advanced that a move to the nursing home may be uneventful and even required due to a need for skilled nursing care at that juncture.

Common sense rule: Weigh Program, Proximity, and Price in selecting care.

Summary

Don't be afraid to ask for and accept caregiving assistance from family, friends, and professionals. Explore options and identify resources as soon as possible. Consider early enrollment in adult day programs (Brain Therapy) to maintain a loved one's social engagement and activity level and provide caregiver relief. Primary family caregivers should utilize respite care provided by relatives, professionals, or others to avoid caregiver burnout. Pick a residential care facility that would best serve a patient in case it might be needed in a crisis situation (e.g., if a primary caregiver falls ill or has to travel). Don't hesitate to move a loved one to the level of care that works best.

Common Sense Rules

- Engage help early and often.
- Identify caregiving options and benefits as soon as possible.
- Be creative and cooperative in helping your loved one with dementia.

- Help the Helper.
- Make a family plan of care.
- The patient may need a break from the caregiver!
- The most expensive choice is not always the best.
- Respite care offers a temporary option to permanent placement.
- Don't delay in finding a facility to best suit the needs of your loved one with dementia.
- Get on the waiting list for the facility of choice.
- Ask questions.
- Don't judge a program by its title (or its décor).
- Know signs indicating the need for supervised and secure living.
- Consider facilities that offer multiple levels of care.
- Make the move to a higher level of care as and when needed.
- Think of Hospice sooner rather than later.
- Weigh Program, Proximity, and Price in selecting care.

Websites

Medicaid information: www.cms.gov
Medicare: www.medicare.gov

References

1. Dubinsky RM, Stein AC, Lyons K. Practice parameter: risk of driving and Alzheimer's disease (an evidence-based review): report of the quality standards subcommittee of the American Academy of Neurology. Neurology. 2000;54(12):2205–11.
2. Iverson DJ, Gronseth GS, Reger MA, Classen S, Dubinsky RM, Rizzo M, Quality Standards Subcomittee of the American Academy of Neurology. Practice parameter update: evaluation and management of driving risk in dementia: report of the Quality Standards Subcommittee of the American Academy of Neurology. Neurology. 2010;74(16):1316–24. Epub 2010 Apr 12.
3. Assisted Living Federation of America. Overview of Assisted Living: a collaborative research project of AAHSA, ASHA, ALFA, NCAL & NIC. Alexandria, VA: Stratton Publishing and Marketing Inc.; 2009.
4. Rosenblatt A, Samus QM, Steele CD. The Maryland Assisted Living Study: prevalence, recognition, and treatment of dementia and other psychiatric disorders in the assisted living population of central Maryland. J Am Geriatr Soc. 2004;52:1618–25.
5. Sloane P, Zimmerman S, Ory MG. Care for persons with dementia. In: Zimmerman S, Sloane P, Eckert JK, editors. Assisted living: needs, practices, and policies in residential care for the elderly. Baltimore, MD: Johns Hopkins University Press; 2001. p. 242–71.
6. van Zadelhoff E, Verbeek H, Widdershoven G, van Rossum E, Abma T. Good care in group home living for people with dementia. Experiences of residents, family and nursing staff. J Clin Nurs. 2011:2490–500. doi: 10.1111/j.1365-2702.2011.03759.x. Epub 2011 Jul 18.

Chapter 16
Looking Ahead: The Later Stages

Worry does not take away tomorrow's troubles. It takes away today's peace.

This chapter addresses the end-of-life decisions that families face for a loved one with advanced dementia. For patients with advanced dementia, we look for a compelling reason to justify additional assessments or interventions. It sounds logical in theory, but can be challenging in practice. The general rule of thumb is not to test for a condition that you're not going to treat. Here is a formula we suggest that you follow in determining whether to proceed with any medical intervention. First, think ahead to what treatment you would reasonably allow. Then, work backwards to decide if any type of assessment, work-up, or diagnostic test is warranted.

Unfortunately, medical care often continues at the same intensity level for a patient with advanced dementia without much thought as to whether this is appropriate. Physicians may be uncomfortable deviating from routine medical care. A patient's relatives may passively follow physician recommendations without realizing that tests, procedures, and other interventions can be declined. And even with awareness of the option to refuse, a family member may have a hard time saying no to further interventions.

Common sense rule: Don't do the test if the result won't change the plan of care.

A.M. Lipton and C.D. Marshall, *The Common Sense Guide to Dementia for Clinicians and Caregivers*, DOI 10.1007/978-1-4614-4163-2_16, © Springer Science+Business Media, LLC 2013

Medical Care in Advanced Dementia

Comfort Care

This should be the principle guiding medical care in advanced dementia. We aim to preserve a patient's quality of life, with an emphasis on relieving, avoiding, or at least minimizing pain and avoiding unnecessary and futile medical tests and treatment. Even transport to a clinic or noninvasive tests may be difficult for such patients.

What do we mean by advanced dementia? In this stage of dementia, patients depend on others for most or all of their basic ADLs, such as dressing, bathing, eating, brushing teeth, etc. Such patients typically have very poor memory and may not remember key information, such as date of birth, where they live, or some family members (particularly those known to the patient for the shortest amount of time, such as grandchildren or new in-laws). They cannot understand or participate in complex decision-making, such as that required for medical, legal, and financial issues. Many will have behavioral problems, such as agitation. At this stage of dementia, patients may be candidates for Hospice Care (discussed in the last chapter and in further detail below), which emphasizes comfort care only.

However, even a patient not eligible for Hospice or whose family (or other medical decision maker) chooses to decline Hospice care may still have comfort care or even comfort care only. The following sections provide some practical approaches for medical care in advanced dementia and may apply to other stages of dementia as well, depending on individual circumstances.

Common sense rule: Comfort care works with or without Hospice care.

Medical Procedures

Let us say your loved one with dementia has an abdominal aortic aneurysm that is being monitored for an increase in size. Such an aneurysm is an abnormal swelling in the aorta, which is the largest blood vessel in the body. Typically, if an aneurysm is found, tests are done to monitor its size for surgical correction if it becomes large enough. The question is whether to keep doing the tests in a patient with advanced dementia. Thinking ahead, if you are the medical decision maker for such an individual and would not consent for your loved one to undergo a major surgery even if the aneurysm is increasing in size, there is no reason for continued monitoring.

Likewise, let us say a patient with advanced dementia has a history of breast cancer and undergoes routine mammograms to look for cancer recurrence. Thinking ahead, if you are the medical decision maker for this patient and would not choose to expose your loved one to chemotherapy, radiation, or surgery, mammograms may be discontinued.

Many families continue to schedule their loved ones with dementia for screening tests out of habit. Take a moment to think through the physical and psychological consequences of such evaluations, which may include mammograms and colonoscopies, blood draws (e.g., for cholesterol checks), and prostate and gynecological exams. These tests may distress anyone, but particularly a patient who does not understand the rationale.

An annual Pap smear is important in screening for cervical cancer, but it requires that a woman disrobe, put her legs in stirrups, and undergo an invasive exam in an intimate area. It makes no sense to subject a woman with advanced dementia to such an evaluation if her family (or other medical decision maker) would not pursue treatment for any cancer found. This logic applies to other screening procedures (e.g., colonoscopies) as well. For patients with advanced dementia who may become agitated and uncooperative with the exam, these tests might even become painful or dangerous.

Sometimes patients with advanced dementia have particular symptoms, including pain, justifying certain procedures, but, even then, the options should be clearly weighed. For example, can the patient's pain or other symptoms be addressed without invasive testing? Is the patient a candidate for Hospice?

Most patients with advanced dementia lose weight, but, in most cases, this may be attributed to late stages of dementia and does not indicate a need for a colonoscopy to look for a cause. Again, if colon cancer were found, would any treatment but pain relief be desired? And, if comfort care is the priority for a given patient, why subject him or her to an invasive test? The bottom line is that the risks of medical screening in patients with advanced dementia may confer no benefit and pose significant risks.

For some patients with advanced dementia, the risks of any disruption to their environment (such as leaving a residence for a clinic) outweigh the potential benefits of any procedure done in which transport is required.

Routine laboratory blood tests (e.g., for cholesterol levels) should generally be avoided in patients with advanced dementia. For those who become agitated, an attempt to insert a needle could injure the patient, the phlebotomist (person drawing blood), or others. If such a patient takes any medications that require blood checks, it may be worth stopping this drug or switching to another that does not necessitate such tests.

Common sense rule: Stop routine medical screening in advanced dementia.

Dental Care

Along the same lines, routine dental cleaning may be discontinued for patients with advanced dementia who may become fearful and overwhelmed by the exam. In case of a compelling reason to intervene, such as a painful tooth abscess, the dentist may recommend anesthesia or other sedation both for patient comfort and staff safety due to risk of biting. In such cases, if the dental procedure is necessary, then such sedation may also be justifiable.

Common sense rule: Discontinue routine dental care in advanced dementia.

Medications

As we discuss elsewhere, regular review of medications benefits patients with dementia. As the disease advances, medical personnel, families, and other caregivers should consider stopping or minimizing medication that may no longer offer more benefit than risk. In addition, families may not want to pursue any treatment that could prolong life. Some may prefer to apply any cost savings to other aspects of a patient's care. Others may just have a "less is more" philosophy.

Terminating a drug (or any medical intervention) is usually psychologically difficult, however, not just for family members, but also for doctors and other medical personnel. It may, nonetheless, be the preferable, or even necessary, option. Therefore, don't start medications without good justification and consider adjustments as a patient's condition changes. This should always be done with medical advice and supervision, particularly from a prescribing physician, and especially because some medicines may need to be withdrawn slowly.

For each medication, ask the questions: (1) What is the reason for taking this drug? and (2) What are the risks and benefits? Discuss these issues with the prescribing doctor to determine whether to (1) continue, (2) stop, or (3) reduce the dosage of medicine.

If a patient's doctor doesn't raise these questions, family caregivers (or other patient decision makers) most definitely should. This especially applies to cases in which a patient has dysphagia (difficulty swallowing) or trouble taking medication regularly for any other reason. A discussion amongst doctors and families can help allay fears and concerns, lead to a careful and considered decision, and bring peace of mind for all.

Routine Medications Unrelated to Dementia

Let's say your loved one with advanced dementia takes a cholesterol-lowering drug. Your family member may have had a prior heart attack, done well on this medication, and you and the patient's physician decide to continue it. However, as dementia progresses, cholesterol, appetite, and/or weight often lessen and may justify stopping this medication. Maybe your family member can no longer cooperate with having blood drawn (or you have decided that he or she should no longer be subjected to such tests). Perhaps the aim of reduced risk of heart attacks and strokes no longer justifies its use due to stage of disease, cost, and/or other factors.

Neuropsychiatric Medications

These treat dementia, anxiety, depression, and other mood and behavioral symptoms.

Dementia medications do not appear to prolong life in Alzheimer's disease [1], and little evidence exists to support such a role in other types of dementia. However, behavioral symptoms may emerge when medicines specifically designed to treat dementia are stopped, even in patients who have no history of behavioral problems or who have not had any in some time [2]. Therefore, these medications may be justified in advanced dementia for reasons of preventing or treating behavioral symptoms, such as agitation.

Non-pharmacologic treatment should be tried for mood and behavioral symptoms which occur despite treatment with dementia drugs. Other neuropsychiatric agents may pose significant risks and should be used judiciously. Chemical and physical restraint of patients should be avoided. For example, medications should be adjusted for a patient who appears overly sedated.

Unless specific new issues arise, we almost always recommend that our patients with advanced dementia stay on the regimen that has worked for them previously. However, it is important to regularly check that the benefits of each medication continue to outweigh the risks.

Stopping one or more of these medicines may be a consideration due to cost or other issues. Dosage reduction may be indicated due to sedation, poor appetite, or other symptoms. If a decision is made to attempt withdrawal or reduction, we highly recommend following the measures discussed in the chapter on medications. Namely, only one medicine should be adjusted at a time, and this should be done slowly, cautiously, and with medical supervision. Any problems arising may then be addressed by restarting the drug or resuming the prior dosage of the drug.

Appetite Stimulants

We do not recommend medications solely prescribed to stimulate appetite in our patients with advanced dementia. Overall, studies of appetite stimulants in dementia show some benefit for weight gain, but not for prolonging life, improving function, or otherwise enhancing quality of life [3]. We therefore look to what medications might be stopped, reduced, or switched in order to maintain health. For example, cholesterol-lowering medication could be discontinued for a patient who is no longer eating much. If a patient has previously done well on an oral form of a cholinesterase inhibitor, but is now experiencing poor appetite and weight loss, this type of anti-dementia medication might be switched to a patch form to minimize these symptoms. For a patient needing a sleep aid, we might try mirtazapine in low doses to stimulate appetite and weight gain. (Note that mirtazapine may also be used to treat mood and behavioral symptoms besides insomnia.)

Common sense rule: Streamline medications.

Consolidated Care

While one or more specialists may benefit a patient in initial stages of dementia, advanced dementia may be the time to consolidate care. Consider conducting all of a patient's care via one physician. First, identify the doctor who will adopt this role and make sure that he or she is comfortable with this plan.

This might be the primary doctor (such as an internist, family practitioner, or geriatrician) who has cared for your loved one for years. If it is difficult to transport your family member to the primary doctor's office, you might ask for a recommendation for a physician house calls service.

A physician affiliated with the long-term-care facility in which your loved one resides could also serve in this role. This doctor visits patients on-site, thus eliminating the need to take your loved one out of the facility for such evaluation. This approach has pros and cons. It may benefit a patient and enhance care by allowing the doctor to examine the individual in a familiar place, easily access the medical chart and medications, and facilitate discussion with nursing and other staff who regularly interact with the patient. Families love the convenience, particularly when it is a struggle to get a loved one out and about. Medical issues and families' concerns can be addressed promptly when they arise. On the negative side, sometimes families don't have as much interaction with the doctor as with a family physician. They may worry that the visiting physician is unaware of pertinent health history, including current issues, particularly when the patient is no longer able to contribute relevant information during an exam.

When considering a doctor affiliated with a facility or who makes house calls, ask if the visiting physician works alone or as part of a team of nurse practitioners or physician assistants, who may see your loved one more frequently than the doctor supervising the care. The latter is the typical arrangement and often works well. If your loved one is enrolled in Hospice, the medical team operates similarly and is yet another option for point-of-care.

In any event, if your loved one currently follows with a primary care physician, have him or her weigh in on the decision. He or she will likely have invaluable insight into the particulars of your loved one's situation (and yours).

Speak with specialists to see if their medications and care can and should be transitioned to the primary care physician and, if so, how best to do this. If a patient has significant psychiatric or behavioral issues, it may also make sense to continue care with a dementia specialist, such as a psychiatrist or a neurologist.

Common sense rule: Consolidate medical care in advanced dementia.

Emergency Room Visits and Hospitalizations

Families often do not realize that they have a say in whether their loved one goes to the emergency room (ER). If a patient with advanced dementia lives at home, family can agree not to call emergency services or send a loved one to the emergency room.

We recommend discussing this with all relevant and concerned family members and doctors and putting instructions in writing to avoid confusion and miscommunication. If a loved one with dementia lives at a facility, you will need to speak with the facility's administrator. The facility may require written documentation of a family's wishes as they may have internal procedures where ER visits are automatically triggered by certain events, such as a fall, fainting, or chest pain. Such visits are usually avoided for patients in Hospice Care, but may be called for in some circumstances. Family members should discuss this with the Hospice medical team. However, even if a patient with advanced dementia is not in Hospice Care, transport to an emergency room doesn't need to occur if the patient's medical decision maker decides against it. Ideally, this decision should be arrived at, documented, and communicated to a patient's doctors and family members well in advance and not in the midst of an emergency situation. And, Hospice Care should be seriously considered for such a patient.

Common sense rule: It is possible to avoid hospitalization in advanced dementia.

Resuscitation Status

If a patient does not have directives in place, family members will most likely need to determine resuscitation status. If resuscitation is not desired, it is best to document this decision in advance of any emergency, since withdrawing care tends to be much more difficult psychologically and emotionally than simply avoiding an unwanted procedure in the first place.

Survival rates of elderly patients after resuscitation are under 10 % [4–6]. Therefore, it is usually difficult to justify subjecting a person with advanced dementia to the rigors of a resuscitation effort.

What Does DNR Mean?

DNR stands for "Do Not Resuscitate." Therefore, Cardiopulmonary Resuscitation (CPR) will not be administered by anyone present or emergency medical services (EMS) will not be called to administer CPR if a patient's heart or breathing stops. All noninvasive, non-painful efforts to make a patient comfortable still can and should be made.

In reality, sometimes EMS are still called in a nonhospital setting (e.g., home, assisted living, rehabilitation or long-term-care facility). This may be due to uncertainty about a patient's medical condition, a facility's policies, etc. If EMS are called, they could be called again and told that they are not needed (however, once en route, they often must proceed regardless). If EMS does arrive, the patient's DNR directive should be produced and shown immediately to them so that they can avoid administering unwanted and unnecessary resuscitation efforts.

DNR forms and regulations vary from state to state. Blank DNR forms may be found online or requested from medical institutions and clinics, including hospitals, doctors' offices, home health agencies, and long-term-care facilities. They generally require the approval and signatures of the person with medical decision-making power for the patient and at least one physician.

What Is Resuscitation?

As its name suggests, CPR includes two basic components: trying to restart a heart that has stopped beating normally and providing oxygen to someone who has stopped breathing normally. One physiologic process can go on independently for a short time, but the two often go hand in hand if no intervention is made. That is, if you stop breathing, your heart soon follows and vice versa.

Resuscitation is generally not gentle and may not best serve the interests of a patient with advanced dementia or other terminal, irreversible illness. CPR may include removing clothing from the upper body, chest compressions (repeatedly pushing down on a patient's chest with both hands using the weight of your own body—this can and sometimes does result in broken ribs), precordial thump (hitting the chest to try and restart the heart), and defibrillation (using paddles to deliver electric shocks, which can cause burns). It may also involve mouth-to-mouth resuscitation to deliver breaths to a patient.

Advanced Cardiac Life Saving (ACLS) resuscitation techniques may be performed outside the hospital by EMS (including ambulance personnel such as Emergency Medical Technicians, also called paramedics) or by nurses and doctors in a hospital or a similar setting. ACLS includes CPR and may also involve putting a breathing tube down a patient's throat and airway (windpipe), inserting an intravenous (IV) line via a needle into a vein (or using a preexisting one) to deliver medications, and other procedures.

As you can see, resuscitation can be painful and invasive. What you might be surprised to learn is, unlike what you see on TV and in the movies, how often it fails, even for patients for whom it is appropriate. CPR administered by medical professionals is successful only 15 % of the time for hospitalized patients [4–6] and less than 10 % for those outside the hospital [7]. Contrast this to fictional television programs and movies in which CPR is depicted as successful more than two-thirds of the time [8]. Therefore, CPR may not only be a rough procedure for a patient with advanced dementia, but also most often will be in vain.

> I'm moving my husband to a memory facility due to his advanced dementia. They asked me about DNR status, since I am his Medical Power of Attorney and his doctor said that he is no longer capable of making his own decisions regarding such matters. I don't know his specific wishes, but I suspect he wouldn't want his life prolonged. He always talked about not wanting to be a burden. However he's in pretty good health. I'm not sure what to do.

First and foremost, try to make the decision that your husband would if he were able and act in his best interests. If you have considered all of the foregoing and your gut then tells you that he would not want resuscitation given his current condition, then you can complete and sign forms to designate his status as "DNR" (usually with the agreement and signature of at least one of his doctors). Provide a copy to the facility and his physicians. It may help to discuss this decision with other family members and doctors or at least inform them of it. It's certainly important to document.

A DNR directive provides a way to protect patients from having to go through possibly uncomfortable, unnecessary, and futile CPR in the last moments of their lives. Such patients can instead be made comfortable via much kinder and gentler measures.

Common sense rule: Doing everything for a patient may not be best for the patient.

Avoid Feeding Tubes

We strongly discourage the use of feeding tubes in dementia. Based on the preponderance of medical evidence [9] which has shown that:
Feeding tubes in dementia:

- Do NOT prolong survival.
- Do NOT decrease the risk of aspiration pneumonia (pneumonia developing when food or saliva goes down a person's airway or windpipe instead of the esophagus).
- Do NOT improve a patient's functional status.

But, feeding tubes in dementia are associated with:

- Increased infection.
- A substantial number of deaths at the time of or shortly after the procedure for tube insertion.

And, in a recent study [10], family members whose loved ones with advanced dementia died with a feeding tube in place were less likely to report excellent end-of-life care than those whose loved ones did not have a feeding tube.

Common sense rule: Avoid feeding tubes for dementia.

Consider Hospice

Hospice evaluation should be strongly considered for a patient with advanced dementia and eligibility for this was discussed in the last chapter. Our families almost universally endorse positive experiences with hospice. In addition to the medical care they provide, hospice team members offer their extensive experience and unique skills to address the emotional and spiritual issues that arise for patients and their families. Several patient families have reported that the greatest blessing of their time with hospice was not feeling alone.

Letting Go, Gently

There comes a point in any illness that we, as physicians and families, need to follow a loved one's lead and let nature take its course.

> I just don't understand it. Mom is clearly ready to go. She would never want to live this way. But she just hangs on. It's so hard to watch.

Wow. This is tough stuff and hard to watch, let alone for family and other caregivers to live through each. Here we have a situation where Mom's body has outlived her mind. At this point, family members may have made peace with a loved one's passing. They may even see Mom's death as a blessing, believing she will go on to a better place. It is important to look at what we (physicians, family, and other caregivers) are doing and see if we are doing anything to actively block a loved one's efforts to go in peace. If DNR status has been designated, we can then move on to whether we should continue to treat medical symptoms and illness. Our health care system defaults to treating almost anything, whether it should be or not. We want to avoid overwhelming the brain further with repeated and futile medical interventions. Are we sending Mom to the emergency room each time she is somnolent, confused, or falls? Are we testing and treating for all medical problems, including every instance of possible dehydration and infection? Answering these questions in the affirmative is not necessarily a good thing, the right thing, or the best thing for a patient with advanced dementia. We need to talk about why we're continuing to utilize the hospital and treating infections, and, most importantly, if we should stop. From a medical standpoint, we might think of simply letting nature take its course. From a philosophical standpoint, we may wish to try and align ourselves with the course the patient is following. You might think of it as following Mom's lead. A spiritual viewpoint might suggest that by blocking Mom's exit from this world, we're blocking the threshold of heaven.

You may consider these and other points of view, but the crux is to find and follow your path alongside your family member. Take comfort in knowing that your loved one doesn't have to go it alone.

Common sense rule: Follow your loved one's lead.

Our parting wish for all who read this book is peace. One of the greatest gifts you can give your loved one is reaching an inner peace about his or her journey, including its end. This is a journey in itself. Discuss it openly with the people who matter to you and your loved one with dementia, including family, friends, and other caregivers. Let go of grudges, guilt, and unresolved issues. Always remember, your loved one will only do as well as you are doing. So, let yourself find and feel at least some serenity. Peace is a gift. Allow yourself to accept it.

Dear Caregiver, we salute you. Thank you for all that you do.

Summary

When evaluating the utility of medical assessments or interventions, use the compelling reason rule: Don't do the test if the result won't change the plan of care. Emphasize comfort and consolidate medical care for patients with advanced dementia. Review and streamline medications. Avoid excessive and futile intervention, such as feeding tubes. Consider palliative care/Hospice care in advanced dementia. Take comfort and find peace and self-worth in your vital role as caregiver and companion to your loved one with dementia.

Common Sense Rules

- Don't do the test if the result won't change the plan of care.
- Doing everything for a patient may not be best for the patient.
- Comfort care works with or without Hospice care.
- Streamline medications.
- Avoid feeding tubes for dementia.
- Follow your loved one's lead.

Common sense rules specific to patients with advanced dementia (but which may be considered in other stages of dementia, depending on individual circumstances):

- Stop routine medical screening.
- Discontinue routine dental care.
- Consolidate medical care.
- It is possible to avoid hospitalization in advanced dementia.
- Consider Hospice.

Websites

Alzheimer's Association: www.alz.org
Caring.com: www.caring.com
Family Caregiver Alliance: www.fca.org
National Hospice and Palliative Care Organization /National Hospice Foundation:
http://www.nhpco.org

References

1. Rountree S, Chan W, Pavlik V, Darby E, Doody R. Factors that influence survival in Alzheimer's patients. Alzheimers Dement. 2011;7(4 Suppl):S513.
2. Holmes C, Wilkinson D, Dean C, Vethanayagam S, Olivieri S, Langley A, Pandita-Gunawardena ND, Hogg F, Clare C, Damms J. The efficacy of donepezil in the treatment of neuropsychiatric symptoms in Alzheimer disease. Neurology. 2004;63(2):214–9.
3. Hanson LC, Ersek M, Gilliam R, Carey TS. Oral feeding options for people with dementia: a systematic review. J Am Geriatr Soc. 2011;59:463–72.
4. Murphy DJ, Murray AM, Robinson BE, Campion EW. Outcomes of cardiopulmonary resuscitation in the elderly. Ann Intern Med. 1989;111(3):199–205.
5. Varon J, Fromm Jr RE. In-hospital resuscitation among the elderly: substantial survival to hospital discharge. Am J Emerg Med. 1996;14(2):130–2.
6. Taffet GE, Teasdale TA, Luchi RJ. In-hospital cardiopulmonary resuscitation. JAMA. 1988;260(14):2069–73.
7. "CPR statistics." American Heart Association. Retrieved 2011-11-1.
8. Diem SJ, Lantos JD, Tulsky JA. Cardiopulmonary resuscitation on television. Miracles and misinformation. NEJM. 1996;334(24):1578–82.
9. Finucane TE, Christmas C, Travis K. Tube feeding in patients with advanced dementia: a review of the evidence. JAMA. 1999;282(14):1365–70.
10. Teno JM, Mitchell SL, Kuo SK, Gozalo PL, Rhodes RL, Lima JC, Mor V. Decision-making and outcomes of feeding tube insertion: a five-state study. J Am Geriatr Soc. 2011;59(5):881–6.

Index

A

Abnormal motor behavior, 139
Acetylcholine reduction. *See* Cholinesterase
    inhibitors (CIs)
Acetyl-L-carnitine, 101
Activities, behaviors, and cognition (ABCs),
    3, 85–86
Activities of daily living (ADLs), 4
Adult day programs, 170–172
Advanced health care directives
    do not resuscitate (DNR) directive,
        159–160
    legal document construction, 159–161
Aggression, 137–138
Agitation, 137
Alcohol
    aluminum and Alzheimer's, 120
    bowel products, 117–118
    dependence, dementia, 113–114
    drug exacerbation, 120
    illicit drugs, 118
    intake, physician advice, 112
    medications adverse to memory, 119
    prescription drugs of abuse
        benzodiazepines, 115
        drug duplication, 116–117
        medication withdrawal, 116
        obstructive sleep apnea, 114
        opiates, 114
        sedatives, 115
        sleep disturbances, 114
    withdrawal, 112
Alternative therapies
    chelation therapy, 105
    dementia prevention steps, 106, 107
    diet, 97–98

nutritional and botanical supplements
    description, 98
    magic bullet phenomenon, 99
    6 O' clock news phenomenon, 99
    quality of life consideration, 99
    risks in, 99
quantitative electroencephalogram, 105
scheduled voiding, 104
stem cell therapy, 105–106
stimulatory therapy, 104
supplements
    acetyl-L-carnitine, 101
    caprylidene/caprylic acid, 101
    choline/lecithin, 102
    coconut oil, 102
    coenzyme Q10 (CoQ10), 102–103
    fish oil/omega-3 fatty acids/DHA, 103
    ginkgo biloba, 103
    huperzine A, 103
    melatonin, 104
    phosphatidylserine, 104
    tramiprosate, 104
vitamins
    B, 99–100
    D, 100
    E, 100–101
Alzheimer's disease (AD)
    cognitive enhancers
        (*see* Cognitive enhancers)
    definition, 2
    dementia signposts, 9–10
    depression, 125
Anticholinergic medication, 119
Antidepressants
    behavioral problems, 144
    mood issues, 127

A.M. Lipton and C.D. Marshall, *The Common Sense Guide to Dementia*
for Clinicians and Caregivers, DOI 10.1007/978-1-4614-4163-2,
© Springer Science+Business Media, LLC 2013

CPSIA information can be obtained at www.ICGtesting.com
Printed in the USA
LVOW111321090713

342048LV00004B/12/P